Successful Leadership in Academic Medicine

Successful Leadership in Academic Medicine

David M. Greer
Boston University School of Medicine

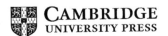

CAMBRIDGE
UNIVERSITY PRESS

University Printing House, Cambridge CB2 8BS, United Kingdom

One Liberty Plaza, 20th Floor, New York, NY 10006, USA

477 Williamstown Road, Port Melbourne, VIC 3207, Australia

314–321, 3rd Floor, Plot 3, Splendor Forum, Jasola District Centre,
New Delhi – 110025, India

103 Penang Road, #05–06/07, Visioncrest Commercial, Singapore 238467

Cambridge University Press is part of the University of Cambridge.

It furthers the University's mission by disseminating knowledge in the pursuit of
education, learning, and research at the highest international levels of excellence.

www.cambridge.org
Information on this title: www.cambridge.org/9781108926294
DOI: 10.1017/9781108923132

First published 2022

Printed in the United Kingdom by TJ Books Limited, Padstow Cornwall

A catalogue record for this publication is available from the British Library.

Library of Congress Cataloging-in-Publication Data
Names: Greer, David M., 1966– author.
Title: Successful leadership in academic medicine / David M. Greer.
Description: Cambridge, United Kingdom ; New York, NY : Cambridge University Press, [2022] |
Includes bibliographical references and index.
Identifiers: LCCN 2021035295 (print) | LCCN 2021035296 (ebook) | ISBN 9781108926294 (paper-
back) | ISBN 9781108923132 (ebook)
Subjects: MESH: Leadership | Faculty, Medical – organization & administration
Classification: LCC RA971.35 (print) | LCC RA971.35 (ebook) | NLM W 21 | DDC 610.69068/3–dc23
LC record available at https://lccn.loc.gov/2021035295
LC ebook record available at https://lccn.loc.gov/2021035296

ISBN 978-1-108-92629-4 Paperback

Contents

Preface

Why do you want to be a leader? Being awarded a leadership position can be considered validation for years of hard work and dedication, an external measuring stick of sorts. Most people in medicine are extremely driven; it takes hard work, discipline, and profound perseverance to succeed in medicine in the first place, even simply to get into medical school. But one quickly realizes that's only the beginning, and the rungs on the ladder become increasingly visible and numerous the more one achieves. Medicine is also incredibly hierarchical – one of my mentors, an organizational psychologist, once told me that medicine was even more hierarchical than the military. I'm not sure I believe that, but then again, I never served in the military. But one glance at academic medicine reveals that hierarchy is not only pervasive – it is likely a *necessary* ingredient to successful care. The levels of leadership are many and diverse, some existing within MD structures (for example, academic teaching services, with attendings, fellows, residents, and medical students), while other paradigms exist for nursing, advanced practice practitioners, and hospital administration. These separate leadership structures often touch each other and overlap, sometimes conflict, and rarely have good knowledge of what the others are doing and prioritizing. This leads to misunderstanding, mistrust, and, potentially, poor clinical care. In short, leadership in medicine is complex and often poorly coordinated. It demands tireless perseverance and sensitive communication skills to navigate frequently challenging situations. Simply put, leadership often entails more than its fair share of headaches and painful situations, and you have to have the stomach for it.

Why *Should* You Want to Be a Leader?

In my opinion, being a leader is about serving others so that the group can be successful. Being a leader is about aligning the goals of the group with the mission, and in medicine, that is often the mission of the hospital/health system/medical school. But the central tenet, which everyone can agree to, is that the patient is at the center of everything we do. "We" can mean the individual or the entire organization; it can mean the clinician, the researcher, or the educator; it can mean the hospital CEO or the greeter or security guard at the front doors of the hospital. We are all there for one goal: to improve the care and lives of our patients, each and every one. This is, of course, stating the obvious, but it's not only important to remember, it's heartening. Consider this your "true north." Being a leader within this structure can be (*should* be) incredibly fulfilling; you can make a difference in people's lives, whether it's the group you're leading, the patients, or both. How many people get to say that their work directly impacts the lives of others in a positive way? It becomes less about the accolades or glory and more about the success of your group and your combined impact on the lives of others.

What Does It Mean to Be a Leader?

There is no such thing as a perfect leader. In fact, if you're chasing perfection, you're sure to be disappointed, and that disappointment will likely affect your performance. It's best to embrace your imperfections and move forward in a positive direction. Surely, working on your weakness is an important part of your growth and development, but also the simple recognition of your weaknesses – even your advertising of those weaknesses to others – may paradoxically make you a more successful leader. Even when a leader is operating optimally, they will inevitably fail to satisfy some portion of the group they lead. This may be due to inherent inequities in the system, limited insight by the leader, or inherent biases in those being led, such that they are naturally inclined to respond adversely to the leader or to leaders in general. Recognize early on that it's not a popularity contest and that your ego is not the most important thing in your leadership role; that title is reserved for the success of those you lead . . . their success as individuals and as a group.

Some like to break down forms of leadership into "servant" leadership, "consensus" leadership, and "authoritarian" leadership. It is convenient to think of these on a spectrum, from the most humble leader to the least. But it's important to recognize that these leadership styles are not mutually exclusive – a single leader can be all three, either at different times depending on the situation or even at the same time! "Servant" leadership implies that the leader is there to serve their constituents, and is a very healthy principle to start with and maintain during one's leadership. The servant leader sees themselves as there to enable the success of others, whether through mentorship, sponsorship, or both (more on mentorship versus sponsorship later). "Consensus" leadership aims to develop consensus among different factions that have competing interests but share a common goal or "roof" (under the umbrella of your domain, typically a department or section). Consensus is not the same thing as agreement; consensus implies that the parties may disagree but have accepted divergent opinions, been respectful of all positions, and have found a way to move forward as a group. "Authoritarian" leadership is as bad as it sounds – the dictator who says, "My way or the highway!" I know of at least one department chair who declared, at his *first* faculty meeting, "This is not going to be a democracy." Not a great way to start your relationship with your new group and hard to backtrack from. But there is a difference between authoritarian and *authoritative*.

In this book, I will walk you through multiple leadership principles, and it will follow a logical progression. First, I will discuss your personal characteristics and motivations for being a leader. We will probe the reasons behind your move into leadership and what personality traits will serve you best – and worst. Next, we'll discuss how you build your team, including establishing a culture and identity and rallying around a mission and vision. Given its importance, an entire chapter will be devoted to "Running an Effective Meeting" – one of the most challenging aspects of a leader's role but crucial to achieving the goals in most groups in medicine. Then, we will dive into how to align your group's goals with the hospital and medical school (for those in academic medicine), an often-overlooked step but one that can greatly enhance the success of your team and increase its longevity and impact. Finally, we'll handle the most challenging aspects of medical leadership – having difficult conversations and leadership in a crisis (this book was written during the beginning of coronavirus pandemic, which taught invaluable lessons to those in medical leadership). We will conclude with a look toward the future – how to truly grow and excel in medical leadership ("Medical Leadership 2.0").

I did not launch into my medical career thinking I would ever write a book on leadership. In fact, I did not enter my medical career thinking I myself would be a leader someday (despite my somewhat famous neurologist father). I fell into leadership slowly and naturally and found I had a great love and passion for good leadership. I had many mentors in my career; some were truly amazing, but some were what I would call "negative mentors" – examples I did not want to emulate. Both types of mentors are helpful, believe it or not, as without the examples of negative mentorship, I would not have been able to define some potential pitfalls or personality traits that would have worked against me. My first leadership position was Residency Program Director when at the Massachusetts General Hospital, and I only applied for the position because the residents encouraged me to do so. Several years later, I was recruited to Yale to become the Clinical Vice Chair, a marvelous position that really taught me the ropes in how to build and run a clinical service – inpatient, outpatient, intensive care, residency, fellowship – and to coordinate with hospital and medical school leadership. It was there that I got the itch, after only a few years, to be a chair myself, motivated not by the glory or glamour that comes with the title but with the realization that I would be more gratified professionally in a position in which I could have greater impact. In 2017, I came to Boston University/Boston Medical Center, a very strong medical school associated with a very strong safety-net hospital, with a storied history in excellence in neurological care, education, and research but also a mission to care for the underserved. The move was a good one; I have never felt more fulfilled or impactful in my career, and I have learned a great deal about medical leadership – both through successes and failures.

One day, I put down a list of 10 leadership qualities that I thought were important and posted them on social media. I'm not exactly sure why, as I'd never posted something like that before and am not a big user of social media. But many of my friends and former residents commented that they were moved by my thoughts, and some suggested I write a book. So here we are! Although there are many books on leadership out there, there are very few on leadership in medicine in particular. Hopefully the discussion in this book is helpful to you, whether you're already a leader in medicine or you're thinking of becoming one. I wrote this with an eye toward practicality, organized in a structure that I thought would be most helpful. I hope it helps you to achieve your goals as a leader but, more importantly, the goals of the group you lead.

Why Do You Want to Lead?

If you're considering a leadership position in medicine, you are not alone. Leadership positions in the field of medicine are plentiful, and given the inherent hierarchies in medicine, it's natural to find oneself tapped to lead one group or another eventually. This does not mean that you will be a good leader or that the leadership position is the right one for you. But not to worry, most often there is another, and another, opportunity, and you usually won't hurt yourself too badly by failing in your first leadership position or even failing to take it. You always have a choice, although sometimes the choices can seem incredibly hard!

Before you take on a leadership position, you should ask several important questions: (1) What is the position, and do you fully understand what it entails? (2) What is your "phenotype" as a leader or, rather, your skill set or areas of strength? (3) Is the leadership position a good "fit," for you and for them? (4) Do you have the desire to lead? Why? (5) What is (are) the next step(s) after this move? Is it a bridge? It could be a bridge to a higher or more appropriate position, or a bridge to nowhere. And it's often difficult to tell at first.

This chapter will set the table for your personal decisions when considering taking a leadership position, and explore what should go into your thinking as you're weighing your options. Keep in mind that, although you may be paralyzed with fear, it is pretty uncommon to make disadvantageous choices when it comes to leadership opportunities, at least early in your career. But the onus is on you to follow through and make the most of the opportunity!

What Is the Position?

Too often, I've seen people get starry-eyed about a potential leadership position. Maybe they weren't expecting to be offered the position, and it may have come as a real boost to their ego. Or perhaps it hit them at the right time, and they were eager to leap at the opportunity. A bit of unsolicited advice: slow down. I would be hard-pressed to think of an instance in which you would need to make a critical decision about a leadership position quickly or under duress, unless it were stepping in on a temporary basis due to extenuating circumstances for a leader who abruptly left the position. Otherwise, you should take your time to gather as much knowledge about the position as possible. If you're considering the role, that's because someone (maybe only you!) feels that you might be worthy of it. But is the position worthy of, or right for, you?

Do your homework. If there is a job description, ask for it. If there isn't a job description, consider whether one could or should be created, and ask for it. In other words, know what you're getting yourself into and what the expectations of you will be. Get as granular as possible – what will be required to do the job, what kind of resources will be made available, what kind of support or team will you be able to assemble? Hand-in-hand with the *work* goes the *time* – if the tasks are large, you will need to clarify how much effort will be required and how much time should be allotted, both in the short and long terms. Will you have protected time to do the job, and will that time be adequate? Are the deliverables reasonable? Do you have a legitimate chance of getting the job done, based on what you find out about what is required?

Consider establishing metrics for your success over time, and make sure that whoever is evaluating your performance agrees with the metrics. If you establish these metrics ahead of time and they're agreed to, it leads to far less confusion down the road and also allows you to recalibrate as you progress or, alternatively, if obstacles set you back. With all this said, however, sometimes there are things that cannot be "metricized" about a job, such as HR issues or dealing with problematic group members. These things become *more* common the higher you go up the food chain, not less. As they say about children, "the older the kid, the bigger the problems." The same applies in medical leadership as well – the egos become bigger as the CVs grow longer, and thus the HR and personality issues become more prominent. The earlier and better you learn to deal with this in your leadership career, the more successful you'll become (see Chapter 8, "Having Difficult Conversations").

If possible and feasible, talk with the person who held the job before you. Hopefully you will get an honest assessment of the position, warts and all. But keep in mind that, if the person left under inauspicious circumstances, you may not get a fair and unbiased assessment of the position, and you'll need to take their comments with that in mind. An example would be the person who has reluctantly agreed to step down after being asked to resign, who may have negative thoughts about the job, their boss, or both. A better situation is when the person leaving the position is rising to a higher or "better" position and might give a more balanced view. Regardless, vetting the position with the person who is leaving it, when possible, can be invaluable. This is the person best suited to probe for information about the most challenging parts of the job, including working with their supervisor or group. You can clarify time and effort commitments and any positive or negative impacts the role had on their career, as well as their morale. Even information from the "negative" person, that is, the reluctant leaver, can be valuable, as this information can provide leads to important questions for others, most importantly, the people considering hiring/promoting you. Rarely will you find a situation in which you get zero valuable information. It's just that sometimes you'll have to take the info with a grain of salt.

I recall a specific instance many years ago in which I was running a search committee looking for a new chair of another academic department. I had a lengthy discussion with the exiting chair about their impressions of the job and what information would be helpful for the prospective candidates for the position. The outgoing chair was feeling wounded; they were leaving before they felt ready, and being asked to step down was an unexpected and unwelcome shot to their ego. The information they provided me consisted primarily of a list of grievances against the administration – how the department's decline was the administration's fault, not the chair's, and that the department deeply loved them and was "devastated" that they were leaving. Despite my efforts to get information about the *department* that would help the next chair, they kept turning the conversation back to themselves. Nevertheless, the conversation was not a complete waste of time, and I patiently procured a few nuggets of information that would indeed prove helpful in future conversations. Probably most helpful among these was actually trying to corroborate their grievances when I met separately with the faculty. Not surprisingly, they were quite vocal about wanting a change, including hiring someone from outside their own department, as they realized they were victims of stagnation and insular thinking. The impressions of the outgoing chair and the faculty were two complementary pieces of the puzzle and really helped me to advise the chair candidates of what the faculty really wanted and needed.

Be unafraid of asking the difficult questions about the job. When you're trying to figure out if the position is right for you, kick the tires a bit. The person/people looking to hire you will probably respect you more for trying to understand the job as well as you can, including asking the crucial (and sometimes uncomfortable) questions about the challenges the job poses, not just for you but for anyone who might be considering it. Understand that there are those out there who would sell you a lemon; have your radar up, and try to sense whether people are being completely open and honest with you. Ask the same questions of multiple different people, and see if you get the same or different answers. If the latter, you need to circle back and get clarification and consistency. If you can't, they may be hiding something from you. The drawback of this, potentially, is that they might be turned off by your asking too many questions, or questions that are too probing or uncomfortable. If you're on the fence about the position, and there aren't drawbacks to *not* taking it, then being choosy is wise. However, if you really want the job, are worried that you might not get it, and sense that you might be pushing too hard, then it might be better to back off and reweigh your options. If it's a very prominent or prestigious position and there are a lot of good candidates, you may find yourself becoming more seller than buyer. Only you can determine how much to push versus when to cave.

Vet your boss. In almost every leadership position, there's still someone above you to whom you'll answer. That person (or people) may be the chair, the dean, the vice president, the CEO, or even the board. Your understanding of this relationship is crucial. Although you don't have to be best friends (or friends at all) with your boss, you should have a clear understanding of each other's needs, clear communication lines, and some degree of trust in one another. Getting information about your potential boss is not always easy, but whenever you can get ancillary information from others who have worked or are currently working with them, you should. At some point, it becomes a leap of faith, but that leap becomes a lot more comfortable when you have the beginnings of trust in your future boss: you believe in their ethics, and your visions and missions are aligned.

I have had some wonderful leadership relationships in my career, likely because I believe most people in medicine are in it for the right reasons, and it's relatively easy to align goals, specifically around the patient. This includes not just patient care but patient-centered (clinical) research and patient-centered education. But remember, medicine is not a haven from people with big egos, and sometimes very successful people can get swept away by their own achievements, their thoughts ending up centered around themselves rather than what's best for the patient/division/department/institution. This is the boss to worry about – blinded by their own sense of self-importance. This leads to selfish decisions, questionable ethics, and, ultimately, the demise of the group and your relationship. I always like to say that the most powerful quality in medicine is humility and the most dangerous is arrogance. Beware the arrogant boss the most!

What Is Your "Phenotype"?

We all have our strengths and weaknesses; we just rarely have insight as to what they are. Before taking any position, you should take a hard look at yourself and gain a strong understanding of what traits make you successful and which ones hold you back or cause you to fall short. Peering into one's character traits comes easier to some than others; it takes an open mind, a willingness to explore, and a great deal of humility. But even the most introspective and self-critical leaders can have blind spots, only uncovered by working with and seeking the feedback of others. This is where the 360 evaluation becomes essential, as well as working with a coach. I will discuss both of these in detail in Chapter 2.

You have to decide if this leadership position will make you happy or ultimately result in greater fulfillment. Some leadership positions are traps or dead ends, perhaps called leadership positions but actually a form of labor to make someone else's life better. Will you actually be given an opportunity to lead, to innovate, to expand your skill set? Does this step follow logically for what you see as your career path? For example, you could head down an administrative pathway, but the position will take you away from your true passion, which may be more clinically, educationally, or research-oriented. Can you actually see the next step after this one? Does it follow logically? Or is this your ultimate goal, which will provide you with the fulfillment you've been craving? Only you can answer these questions. And your mind may change over time, and that's okay. What you saw as your career goal, such as being a residency program director, may get trumped by a higher position that becomes available to you *because* you became a successful program director.

Consider the push and the pull. To clarify, the pull is the job you're considering taking, and the push is why you're considering leaving your current position. We've talked a bit about what might attract you to a position, but what's the reason you're considering leaving your current one? Once you've vetted your potential new position, it's wise to consider vetting your current position in the same way: what opportunities is the current position providing? What is your relationship like with key people, particularly your boss? Are you growing and developing, and in ways that are helpful to you in the long run? Are you unhappy and running *from* a position, rather than *toward* another one? This is perhaps one of the most important motivations to be aware of, that you may be overly willing to compromise on a new position because you're so eager to leave what you consider a bad situation. Sometimes the "push" is rather strong.

On the other hand, are there negatives to leaving your current position that you've not fully considered? What about the team you're leaving behind – will they feel abandoned or that you've been disloyal by leaving earlier than promised? Have you finished the main parts of the job that you originally signed up for? Are you leaving the group better than when you found them, or are you leaving a trail of destruction? Your reputation will follow you a long way, so it's important to consider what will be said about you after you leave. If you have a reputation as a builder of programs and a good mentor to your people, your reputation will continue to propel you. Alternatively, if your reputation was one of selfishness and using positions and people as stepping stones to higher positions, it will likely come back to haunt you at one point or another.

Consider your individual constraints, including your time and other commitments, both professionally and personally. Leaders commonly bite off more than they can chew, powered by a sense of invincibility, or perhaps just drive and optimism. But we all have limits, and so do the people in our lives. How will the new position impact your ability to tend to other important goals in your life? Your ability to work on that research project, design that new curriculum, or set up that new clinical program? And how about your personal life – will the new position impact your family time or your ability to do self-care such as exercising or relaxing? Does the new position involve a change of location, in addition to hours, and if so, will your partner/spouse/children be negatively impacted? All of these issues must be balanced when you're considering a new position.

Is It a Good "Fit"?

The notion of "fit" is a very visceral one, and it can be challenging to put reasonable metrics to it. In the end, it's still worth trying to do so – at the very least, you can develop a "pro versus con" list that you can utilize in order to provide some degree of objectivity. But it's also good to realize that the "gut" or "gestalt" about a position is important; in fact, it may supersede the objective metrics you've created. If nothing else, the "good vibes" that you have about a position will allow you to carry positivity into the new role, which will likely lead to early successes; conversely, if you're feeling hesitant or less than excited about the new position, you may come off as uncommitted or uninterested, getting you off to a bad start.

When trying to establish your pro and con metrics, remember to do so not just for the leadership position(s) you're considering but also for your current position. That may sound silly, as you probably feel like you already know your current position inside and out, but the process of objectifying it can be very helpful as you force yourself to take a critical look at what you've been doing and what makes you happy versus what does not. One of the "columns" in addition to "pro" and "con" should be "growth potential," assuming you're interested in that. Does your current job contain growth potential? If so, is it growth in the right direction for your overall career goals? Can you get a good estimate for the growth potential of the leadership job you're considering? Be explicit with those looking to hire you – what do they see as your growth potential, both personally as well as in this position? And is there room for growth beyond this position? Again, only you can decide how much you want to grow and climb the ladder, but it's good to have doors opened rather than closed.

The "pros" column in medical leadership positions can contain such things as clinical experience, education, research, or administration, or even other things like mentorship, wellness, work–life balance, and productivity. The "cons" column may contain some of the same issues, but there's often one main difference – we tend to put difficult or painful people in the con category. Each job will be a mix of people that you'll need to work with, both "good" and "bad," and there is no such thing as greener grass. And of course, rarely are people purely good or bad, but rather, their personalities, values, or quirks may work better or worse with *your* personality (and values and quirks). As much as you take a hard look at the people around you, take that same hard look at yourself and understand what you're bringing to the table, warts and all.

Then comes the gut feeling, or as we say in Yiddish, the "gestalt." What does the position/place/people "feel like" to you? What are your emotions after visiting the place, talking with the people, walking the grounds? Objective criteria start to wash away a bit, and the physical space starts to etch itself into your fibers. Do you love the town/city where the job is? Do you like the physical space? Does it feel like "home" in some way? You might walk away thinking that the physical space has made an outsized impression on you, more than it should have, but recognize that the physical space is where you gel your impressions from speaking with the *people*. In fact, it is likely that it was the people all along who were creating your impression. Of course, everyone is putting on their best face when they're trying to recruit you for the position, but you can also get a sense of their genuineness. This also comes with more experience – the more you look at positions, the better your "BS-meter" becomes. Try talking with people who are not on your interview list, such as the staff who work in the area to which you might be hired – the residents, the students, the environmental services people. What do they say about the place? Do they seem happy?

Finally, try to gather a sense for the mission of the place you're considering. Mission can take many forms – some are research heavy, some more geared toward education, others community service-based. None of these missions is "better" than another; it's simply a matter of what fits for your phenotype, and what you're looking for at that stage in your career. For example, a talented physician-scientist may be highly attracted to a leadership position that might lead to a major advance in their lab's capabilities, or at an institution where the philosophy is heavily biased toward generating great basic science research. A different leader might be very drawn to a safety-net hospital that cares primarily for the underserved or has a strong community outreach or global health program. Whatever the emphasis, it has to fit with *your* career goals and motivations, not someone else's.

Do You Have a Desire to Lead? Why?

With leadership positions comes great responsibility. Remember, successful leadership is about the success of the people you're leading, not just your own personal achievements (unless you're a very arrogant and selfish person!). Before taking any leadership position, you have to ask yourself what your motivations are. I'd like to think that people in medicine are generally altruistic and that they carry this altruism with them to their leadership positions. If that desire to "help people," which we all write about in our medical school essays, remains central as you start climbing the medical ladder, then hopefully it can be a guide to what kind of leader you'll be. Sure, there is prestige that comes with leadership positions, and this grows with each rung of the ladder. But you likely won't last very long in most leadership positions if you don't make it about your group and the group's success. Leadership takes sacrifice, both of time and energy, and may take you away from some of the things (for example, research, productivity) that earned you the leadership position. But usually the expectations of you change with the position as well, and in medicine most often the priorities are for the success of the team, not any one individual. In summary, take a hard look at your motivations before launching into any leadership position. You owe it to yourself but, more importantly, to the people you're about to lead.

What Is the Next Step(s) after This? Is It a Bridge (to Nowhere?)?

Like chess, your career moves may dictate subsequent moves, so it's helpful to try to see several moves ahead, if possible. Of course, the position you're considering may be your last stop, or "best stop," but especially if you're junior, you need to think of what will happen to you in five or ten years in this job: will it continue to give you the satisfaction and happiness you desire? This is perhaps one of the hardest things to do when you're considering an upward move – looking past that move to make sure that it will give you long-term fulfillment. Make sure that the new role will give you *more* options in the future, not fewer, as you may not have a clear idea what your ultimate career or leadership goals are; even if you do, they may change over time. So it's always better to open a larger number of doors than end up pigeonholed.

An example of a role that can open more doors for you would be in the realm of education, such as serving as chief resident, clerkship director, or residency program director. All of these roles are typically filled by people with good leadership potential, a strong emotional quotient (EQ), and usually a passion for education and giving of their time to others. With the higher leadership roles (clerkship or residency program director), you're often also seen as someone with education "chops," an expert in some aspect of your field. As you flourish in this educational role and are seen as a good and selfless leader, you are recognized more and tapped for other departmental and institutional leadership roles, such as education vice chair or an associate dean role. Thus, doors are opened.

An example of a role that could be a dead end might be leading a small subcommittee that takes up a considerable amount of your time but does not lead to much recognition or tangible results, a "bridge to nowhere." You need to analyze the amount of time required for the role, the support you'll receive, the timeline, and the expected results; if these don't show promise, you may be wasting your time or, worse, be seen as a failure for not leading the project successfully. Departmental or institutional leadership often has many small committees that need volunteers and leaders, and, without any malice, some of these committees have a low likelihood of success or accomplishment despite best intentions. These are the "buyer beware" proposals that you need to vet to ensure they're right for you, at the right time in your career.

Now that you've done a good self-evaluation, thought about your motivations for wanting to be a leader, and decided on the right position and trajectory, it's time to get into the next steps: understanding your personality as a leader. Although leaders often spend a great deal of time trying to mold their group into their idea of "functional," the molding should actually start with oneself, understanding what personality traits and tendencies you bring to the group that will have a heavy influence on the group's success. Even if you're soft-spoken, you're about to pick up a megaphone. You need to learn how to use it wisely.

Understanding Your Personality as a Leader

Central to running an effective team is knowing your own personality, the good parts and the bad. It is reassuring to know that there are no perfect leaders in medicine, just like in any field, no matter how good some leaders *think* they are. We all have inherent personality traits that can make us more, or less, effective. These are different from "quirks" or "mannerisms" – your personality traits are characteristics unique to you that lead you to think or act in certain ways in a given situation. Some traits we are very aware of and may even use to our advantage (or lament their appearance when unwanted or uncontrollable). Others we are not so aware of, and usually these are more damaging, forming "blind spots" that may push others away, lead to ridicule, or negatively impact the success of the team or project.

Thus, it is essential to take a hard look at yourself and understand your own personality as a leader (or potential leader). The more aware you are of how you act, think, and behave, the more successful you'll be. Keep in mind that this does *not* mean that you will be eliminating these personality traits or changing who you are as a person; it simply means an awareness, so that you can mediate negative effects, accentuate positive ones, and navigate difficult team situations with healthy self-awareness and likely greater success.

What Are Your Strengths?

Now is not the time to be overly humble – most leaders will have some sense of what makes them successful and might make them a good (or great) leader. However, there's a good chance you're not aware of where some of your strengths lie, or your lack of confidence blinds you to potential strengths. A 360 review – seeking feedback from your supervisors, your peers, and your subordinates (if you have them) – can be helpful to gain insight as to how others perceive you, and although we often focus on our weaknesses when we look at 360s, there's great value to looking at our strengths as seen through the eyes of others. Well-designed 360s do a good job of pointing out both the "good" and the "bad." Once you have a clearer idea of your strengths, you can capitalize on them to make yourself more successful as a leader.

Some examples of strengths are listed below. Keep in mind that these are not mutually exclusive, and all leaders have some of these strengths in varying degrees.

- *Charisma.* Some leaders are uniquely inspirational, often due to the charisma they bring when they interact with others. People often look to leaders to have charisma and positivity, even in the worst of times and especially when the team is feeling dejected or failing in a given situation. The charismatic leader can be there to show people where their bootstraps are and how to pull them up.

- *Listening.* This is one of the most commonly touted characteristics of good leaders, that they are good listeners. However, most leaders are not good listeners, often leading to their failure. Those who can truly listen (or at least create the impression that they're actively listening) are often seen as the most effective or caring leaders. And of course, the listening is much more than creating impressions – learning to utilize and incorporate the diverse thoughts of others is key to idea generation and consensus building.

- *Fairness.* Do not underestimate the importance of this! Everyone you lead is frequently (constantly!) looking for signs of fairness in you and will be hypersensitive to slights or impressions of favoritism toward a person/group, especially in your early tenure as a leader. As you establish your track record for fairness, people tend to question it less and trust you more. But make no mistake – saying you're a fair leader does not make you one.

- *Bravery.* Sometimes leaders need to make difficult decisions, including those that will definitely be unpopular with some members of the group. Sometimes a leader needs to jump into the fire and show great leadership at their own potential peril. An example would be a physician leader during a pandemic who leads from the frontline, putting themselves at risk along with other frontliners. This buys you credibility – you have walked the walk in addition to talking the talk, and people take notice.

- *Transparency.* When you do need to make those difficult, often unpopular decisions, if you are transparent about your decision-making, showing people that you've thought out all the options and why you've chosen a specific path, you're much more likely to have buy-in from your group. Sure, some may be unhappy with the decision, but at least they'll know what went into it, which helps whether or not they agree with it.

- *Organization.* Often overlooked, strong organizational skills are essential to good leaders. Some are fortunate to work with an assistant (or multiple assistants) who are able to help them be organized, but even then, there is a learning curve between you and your assistant, and everyone needs to understand the importance of triaging certain appointments or meetings, as well as organizing "self-care" times, such as for exercise and sleep (yes, those are very important!).

- *Humility.* Yes, I listed bravery and charisma above, but again, these are not incompatible with humility. As I said in the last chapter, the most dangerous characteristic in a clinician is arrogance, and the most powerful is humility. When people see you admit your mistakes or shortcomings publicly, it is disarming for them and makes you more approachable and human. They will be *more* willing to follow you, not less, if you let your guard down a bit and show some humility.

- *The three Ps – patience, positivity, and perseverance.* These are my guiding light as a leader. If you're a negative person, you're very unlikely to succeed as a leader (as well as unlikely to be asked to be a leader). If you're unable to persevere through difficult times, you'll likely be a short-lived leader, at least for that position. Patience is often the hardest one, at least for me. But allowing a situation to evolve naturally, when there is no inherent time pressure, is almost always the best course; this allows others to feel unrushed, listened to, and respected. Snap judgments are tempting, and sometimes decisions do need to be made quickly; most often, however, a little patience will bring into focus the right path forward.

Let's shift now to finding out about your weaknesses. A warning: this may be a bit more painful, but it's probably one of the most valuable things you can do as a leader.

Your Weaknesses (and How to Find Them)

Not many people like to talk about their weaknesses, much less hear about them from others. But developing an awareness of your weaknesses is crucial to taking positive steps as a leader. However, it is a step that many are unwilling or unable to take, due to fear, insecurity, or arrogance. But I will argue that it is the most important step in your development as a leader and will give you invaluable insights that can make you and your team highly effective.

So, how do you get the information you need? Self- and others' assessments. The self-assessment is a great place to start and allows you to take a hard look at yourself, answer questions about yourself honestly, and then use this as a comparison for what others say about you regarding the same characteristics. When others agree with you about what you see as your own shortcomings, that is strangely empowering and validating. I personally found it very useful to find out that others saw my limitations in very much the same light that I did, knowing I was not far off base, at least in certain characteristics. But far more useful is the information from others that is different from your own impression of yourself: these are the "blind spots" that need uncovering and will serve as the most important areas for growth and introspection in the future.

There are multiple personality tests available, and most are now administered online. My favorite is the Myers-Briggs Type Indicator (MBTI), which has its origins in the 1940s (www.mbtionline.com). The MBTI roughly distinguishes between certain personality traits or tendencies, although it has come under significant criticism for its lack of validation over the years. Four broad categories emerge: extraversion (E) versus introversion (I); sensing (S) versus intuition (N); thinking (T) versus feeling (F); and judgment (J) versus perception (P), leading to 16 possible combinations or "types." Many of us group into broad categories, such as ESTJ or INFP, but in reality, most of us are not dramatically off to one end of the spectrum or another, and we may even have different qualities at different times or in different situations. I have found that the most dominant characteristic is whether one is an introvert or extrovert, although both can exist within the same individual, and neither makes a better (or worse) leader than the other.

Other available tests specifically evaluate your tendencies as a leader. The DISC Personality Profile (www.discpersonalitytesting.com) is based on William Moulton Marston's DISC theory, which compares and contrasts four distinct styles: Dominance (D), Influence (I), Steadiness (S), and Conscientiousness (C). It is a 28-question assessment designed to give insight into your personality and stylistic tendencies, which may help with your communication style and the overall success of your team.

However, these formal personality tests don't actually get at your weaknesses but rather the personality traits or tendencies that may or may not lead to actual weaknesses. How does one define "weakness" as a leader? Perhaps a useful definition might be a characteristic that leads to poor decisions, poor team rapport or function, or lack of trust, either in the team or in you personally as the leader of the team. Uncovering and truly understanding your weaknesses may come with the use of 360s or a coach or both. We will talk about each of these next.

The Value of 360s

I cannot overstate the importance of 360s in leadership development. But there are several important principles that will ensure you get the feedback you need, and from the right sources. You'll also have to mentally prepare for how you read, interpret, and incorporate the results.

Principle #1: Get a large n. If you get too small a sample size, you'll likely get skewed or only flattering feedback. Most lists of possible evaluators for 360s that are submitted from my faculty are very short – five or ten names at most and filled primarily with people that likely have a favorable opinion of them. It's quite tempting to "stack the deck" with those who you think will tell you you're doing a great job just the way you are, but that defeats the purpose of getting a 360 in the first place. You need a large number of people to evaluate you, and the more the better! You will be tempted to try to figure out "who said what" about you; that's human nature. However, if you get 20, 30, or 50 people to fill out your 360, not only does that become less easy to do, but the temptation also lessens. Furthermore, the aggregate data from a larger number of sources will give you more reliable results when looking at scaled (e.g. Likert) response averages, giving you a truer picture of your scores on more standardized questions. These scores, although somewhat subjective, are still more objective than free-form written responses (although I'll argue that the latter can be just as valuable, if not more). Plus, keep in mind that not everyone will fill out your survey; most well-designed 360s take time to fill out, and you'll lose some due to attrition, time, or a desire not to hurt your feelings. Or all of the above.

Principle #2: Solicit 360s from people with whom you don't necessarily have the best relationship. I know this sounds counterintuitive: why would you get people who don't "like" you to fill out a 360 about you? Sounds like asking for insults, right? Well, most of the time, at least in medicine, most people who we *think* don't like us simply have other agendas or might even "like" working with you if they could tell you the things about your personality that make it harder for them. They might be flattered or even excited to know that you valued their opinion enough to solicit it from them in a 360, especially if they know you specifically asked for them. This is their big opportunity to tell you how they "really" feel, and most of the time they'll do so in an honest and direct way. If they end up railing on you, perhaps you can discount it and write it off as the ravings of an angry person. But chances are that they'll give you some of the most useful feedback. That's certainly been the case for me – when I've asked for input from rivals or people with whom I felt I had a less than optimal relationship, it has always been the most useful feedback. But you have to be able to take it. That leads to principle #3.

Principle #3: Put yourself in the right mindset to read your 360 feedback. Here's where your individual personality really figures in – are you the kind of person who craves feedback, whether positive or negative, or are you the kind of person who cringes, avoids, or is downright terrified to hear anything negative? Perhaps you didn't want the feedback at all, but your boss/supervisor thought it was a good idea? And now you're stuck with this *thing* in your in-box that you don't want to open? Some people will build it up into this bigger and bigger *thing*, to the point where they're paralyzed with fear of what it might say and might not even look at it at all.

Perhaps start framing your mindset from the time you come up with your list of assessors, not at the time you're about to open the results. As you're thinking of this person or that, it's healthiest to develop a curiosity or true interest in what they might say about you and what you might learn from them. And remember, the vast majority of feedback about you is likely to be positive! Why do I say this? Because, for the simple reason that you're in (or are being considered for) a leadership position, obviously you've got *some* good qualities. The 360s are about helping you to be better, to develop more insight into yourself and your character, so that you can improve. The natural tendency is to focus on the negative comments or scores, but, depending on your personality, maybe the better place to focus first is on all the things you did well, the qualities that drew people to you and made you an effective leader. Then you can focus on the constructive criticism, once you've built up your confidence a bit.

Regarding the "negative" or critical feedback, I like to use the word "embrace" – if you can embrace the feedback for what it is usually meant to be – anonymized pearls of insight – you're much more likely to read it in the vein intended: to be helpful to you! I would also suggest reading it through several times; your emotions are likely to run high the first time, as no one likes to hear negative things about themselves, at least at first. But if you read it through a second and third time, you may realize that the comments are actually very helpful. You may or may not agree with them, but at least you'll see another point of view, which can be incredibly valuable. A blind spot wouldn't be a blind spot if you could see it.

Principle #4: Process the results! I suggest discussing your results with someone else, preferably a coach or another trained professional, so you can talk through the difficult stuff and come out the other side with a game plan for change, or at least insight. Consider how your evaluators' insights differed from your evaluation of yourself – did you have adequate insight into your shortcomings? Did you rate yourself higher (or lower) than others rated you? If so, why? That in itself can give you tremendous perspective. Were you being completely honest with yourself when you filled out your own 360? Are you over- or underconfident about your abilities? Were the criticisms levied on you accurate, and did you see them yourself, or were they completely out of the blue? Again, this is the holy grail (at least one of them) in your growth as a leader – gaining insight into your strengths and weaknesses in a way that helps you strengthen or adjust your approach to make you more effective and helpful to others.

Getting a Coach (Short and Long Term)

I've had the great fortune of having an amazing coach for many years. But to be honest, it was pure luck. Finding the right leadership coach is quite like finding the right psychologist or psychiatrist – the person may have the best reputation in the world, but if you don't have good chemistry together, it won't work. As you're working on finding the best coach for you, it's best to keep an open mind and try a few people out. It may take a few sessions to know if it's going to work for you or not, and don't be afraid to jump back into the pool of coaches to find the right one if you find that you're not gelling with the current coach. There's no point in staying in the "relationship" if it's not working out – you're paying for a service, it's not the same as dating!

In terms of background, the best coaches for leaders are people with education or training in organizational psychology. One coach once told me that medicine is more hierarchical than the military. I've never been in the military but at least according to this coach, medicine has an inherent hierarchy that may be intensely rigid, often to the point of being dysfunctional. Understanding how all of the moving pieces fit in the hierarchy takes skill and a deep understanding of organizational structure. Most leaders don't have much of an understanding of this, but a good coach should be able to make you aware of this structure and help you to navigate it. Remember, no matter where you are on the food chain, there is always someone else to answer to; even the hospital president answers to the board of directors, and the medical school dean to the university president. Having an understanding of where you fit within the leadership structure of your institution is essential to your success as a leader. You've probably heard the expression that you have to "manage up and manage down" – you must be skilled at both. And sideways (with your peers).

Your first exercise with your coach is likely to be your 360 evaluation. This allows them to gain an understanding of your strengths and weaknesses, both in your eyes and in the eyes of others. They can also help you to process the results of the 360 in a "healthy" way, exploring the areas of discrepancy between your impression of yourself and that of others. Most importantly, they can help you process whatever negative or critical comments you might receive. I love the word "process" here; it's not like putting all of the comments into a blender and coming up with some kind of feedback smoothie – you process the positive and negative feedback differently, and, particularly with the negative, you learn to incorporate the feedback in ways that make you a more effective leader. But that usually takes the expertise of others, and they can also help you overcome the inevitable hurt of the critical comments. Again, if you see the negatives as creating wounds that need to be healed, you're missing the point. They are pearls of insight that help you to grow and learn. You have to process them.

Why does the critical feedback hurt? My coach explains that it's because it touches on a "vulnerability." We all have vulnerabilities, and we often have insight into them, at least subconsciously. That subconscious insight is what causes your emotional reaction. If you thought the comment was inaccurate or did not pertain to you, it would not "hurt." It wounds because there's some truth to it – maybe not complete truth, but enough truth that it stings when you read it, as you recognize that they can see through your armor a bit to a place that makes you "weaker" or less effective as a leader. Well, guess what? They've done you a favor; they've pointed out the chink in your armor so that you can address it. If it didn't hurt a little, it wouldn't have value.

Then comes the reckoning. You and your coach agree on the vulnerability. The next question is "Why?" What is it about you that causes that specific vulnerability? Usually the answer is deeper than you think, and although I don't want to get into psychoanalysis here, some deep probing may be necessary for you to understand why you act in the way you do in certain circumstances, in ways that make you less effective. Maybe these circumstances cause you to lose your cool, or clam up and withdraw, or say things you later regret. You walk away from these interactions with some mixture of anger, frustration, and remorse, often not knowing why. But you know there's something wrong, and most often it may be convenient to blame it on another person (or people) in the room. But it takes two to tango, and you bear some responsibility for every leadership interaction. You may not be able to fully control the situation or conversation, but you can control your reaction to it, and your interactions in the moment.

Short of doing psychoanalysis with your coach, you can use specific case examples to discuss and explore a meeting or interaction that you found problematic. As a leader, your schedule is usually rife with meetings, so there should be plenty of interactions to choose from! I would recommend writing down what you can remember shortly after a suboptimal meeting, so that you can refresh your memory and give a clearer example when you speak with your coach later on. It's especially important to take note of what was said to you that pressed your buttons, what you said in return (particularly things you regret saying), and what you were feeling at the time. Later, when you're with your coach, you can better dissect what happened, why you reacted the way you did, and how your thoughts and feelings got in the way of a better interaction/outcome.

As a specific example, let's say as chair of my department I meet with my hospital administrator to propose a new position, a neuropsychologist to support our dementia program. This seems like an easy sell to me – dementia is a huge public health burden, every neurology department needs to have a dementia program, we need to stay competitive with our local rival hospitals with strong dementia programs, and a neuropsychologist is an essential team member who can best outline cognitive issues and guide therapies. This should not be controversial. The hospital administrator, however, has other thoughts and says (in classic hospital administrator lingo), "Boy, resources are really tight this year, and I don't think we're going to have the bandwidth to support this project in its current state." You leave the meeting frustrated, growling to your department administrative director about how the hospital administrator "doesn't get it," or they're "heartless" and "don't care about the patients." All of these are most likely untrue, but it's easy to fall into the trap of blaming the folks with the money when they don't come through for you.

But who didn't come through? Was it the hospital administrator or you? And why did it sting so much and cause you such frustration? Well, perhaps it was because you failed, and most leaders don't like failure very much! Your coach will help you see that, and moreover, that your failure was due to your lack of preparation. You failed to provide a coherent business case, to help the hospital administrator understand the potential short- and long-term benefits to hiring the neuropsychologist and to the program, such as increased technical revenue, more downstream revenue in the form of neuroimaging, or better outcomes for your patients, always important in hospital advertising. Alternatively, if some of the funding comes from the medical school, the problem may have been failure to show downstream effects such as better educational opportunities for PhD or medical students, or more rigorous research productivity and grant funding. It stings because you should have known better: there is a way to get from point A to point B in medicine, and although you won't always get the funding or the program you need, the bad news will sting less if you know you've done your homework and made your strongest case. The point is, your vulnerability was your embarrassment in your failure to prepare adequately, not the failure to get the funding you needed for the position.

Your coach is a good short- and long-term investment. In the short term, you can have remarkable gains in terms of insight into your character and vulnerabilities, entering a very steep part of your growth curve. But the long term is remarkably valuable as well; your coach has grown to know you well, and you them in return. You have developed trust and compatibility, and even a bit of mind reading, as often happens with couples together for years. You can dig into the heart of the matter much more quickly, as you don't have to rehash most of your prior lessons learned and can swiftly attack and discuss the new issue at hand. You can also use your coach to help with larger projects, such as developing chemistry within your team, holding retreats, and doing personal maintenance and self-checks. One of the most remarkable moments with my coach was when he asked me to list the most valuable or important aspects of my life. I quickly rattled off: (1) family, (2) friends, (3) work, and so on. He then said, "Where is your health on that list?" I hadn't thought of that and responded, "Well, I think it's a given, right?" His response nailed me to my seat: "If you don't make your health your number one priority, you don't get any of the other things on your list." At the time, I was driving myself, at work and at home, extremely hard, and it was affecting my physical health and mental well-being. Prioritizing my health and wellness was exactly what I needed to hear. But I needed someone else to tell me, and thankfully I had my coach there to put things in perspective.

Coursework

There are a vast number of leadership courses available, and I'm not here to endorse one over another. The coursework can take the form of readings about leadership, online courses, or in-person courses. Again, find what works for you. You may be the kind of person who likes to devour literature on leadership concepts from a wide range of authors and formats. Many like the *Harvard Business Review* for relatively shorter, thematic pieces on leadership styles and lessons. Some prefer books on leadership, and two that I like to recommend are *Leading with the Heart* by Mike Krzyzewski (Coach K), the longtime men's basketball coach at Duke University, and *The Five Dysfunctions of a Team* by Patrick Lencioni. I've also long been drawn to biographies (like my father before me), and it can be incredibly helpful to see how some historical figures – Abraham Lincoln, Winston Churchill, and Theodore Roosevelt, to name a few – have handled adversity. Finally, a must read that I always recommend is *The Boys in the Boat* by Daniel James Brown, which combines the principles of leadership and teamwork, as well as the ability to overcome extreme adversity.

In terms of online or in-person courses, certainly word of mouth can be helpful, but make sure to make up your own mind based on the course descriptions as to whether it's the right course for you at the right time in your career. I attended a highly recommended two-week intensive course for new chairs at a major university's school of public health. Although most of my colleagues raved about it, my experience in the end was quite mixed. Pluses included being thrown into an environment with chairs from different medical specialties from all around the country, forming networks and seeing different perspectives. The small-group problem-solving sessions we did were interesting and instructive, not only forcing us to solve the problem at hand but also to work together with other leaders, some of whom had remarkably strong personalities (not always a good thing!). However, minuses included an oppressive reading list (or homework), which was truly impossible to keep up with after a full day of classes and activities, especially since I also had to keep up, as best as possible, with email and small "fires" in my fledgling department. Being away from my "day job" for two weeks was difficult and stressful, and taking the two-week intensive course was far from vacationing or invigorating. I came back exhausted, overwhelmed, and unsure of exactly what I'd learned. Probably most disappointing was the lack of practical advice the course provided for such common problems as dealing with challenging people within your department, which I would have thought to be a primary focus.

In the end, had I been a bit more critical in my homework about the course rather than just taking it because I was told it was "great" and the hospital was paying for it, I might have picked another venue or course that better suited my needs, personality, or long-term goals.

Assessing and Reassessing Your Effectiveness

Effective leadership requires constant and consistent growth, adaptation, and introspection. Your team will rally behind you more (not less) if you are open and welcoming of feedback and criticism. But they need a mechanism to give you that feedback, as well as the knowledge that they won't be the only one doing it and that it may be bidirectional. To make it easier, you can make the feedback anonymous or given as a group. Some may be more comfortable, surprisingly, giving you the feedback directly. You might also structure the feedback as for the team as a whole, rather than for any given individual; even better, you can center it around a group of tasks so that it is not personal to any individual, including you.

I've found the "Stop, start, continue" paradigm to be quite helpful in this realm. As you list out the tasks and objectives of the group, you can ask three simple questions: (1) What is working? (Do more of this.) (2) What is not working? (Do less of this.) (3) What is okay but could be better? (Continue but consider tweaking.) Breaking it down like this can get people to come out of their caves and tell you what's really needed for the project(s) to move forward, and what's holding them back. If you're looking for personal feedback, you can frame like this: (1) What am I doing well? (I should do more of this.) (2) What am I not doing so well? (Consider stopping this, or at least doing a deep dive and revamping the approach.) (3) What am I doing okay, but could be better? (Keep going, but tweak with input.) If you never ask the questions, you'll likely never get the insight to grow and respond to your group.

Finding and Establishing Your (New) Peer Group

As the saying goes, "It's lonely at the top!" When you establish yourself in a new leadership position, you are naturally leaving behind a group of your peers/friends, and it is challenging and often conflicted to maintain the same relationship with them as before. There is now a hierarchy, no matter how much you tell others "not to worry about that." You are now a leader, and they naturally see themselves as answering to you and being subject to your direction. It's not a good thing or a bad thing, just a thing. But your relationship has changed, sometimes dramatically, and it's important to find new peer groups as you rise into different leadership positions, whether you stop at this particular rung or keep climbing. Keep in mind that, as you continue to rise, the peer group gets smaller and smaller. If you rise from resident to chief resident, you will still have lots of peers in your hospital (other chief residents) and at other institutions, as well your program director(s), who are always there to provide support and guidance. As you rise from division chief to vice chair or chair, your peer group has shrunk to vanishingly small, and it's easy to feel isolated and alone.

On the bright side, as you've climbed up the ladder and experienced this sense of isolation and vulnerability, others who have climbed to this same level are almost always experiencing the same thing, or if they've been in the role for a while, they can recall what it was like going through the process initially and can serve as a mentor or guide. For the specific example of chairs, I've found it exciting and invigorating to band together with other chairs to form a new peer group, and I've worked hard to create a functional group that can honestly and effectively discuss problems and ideas and come up with creative and fruitful solutions. I've also found great value in having other, more senior chairs serve as my mentors; my two chair mentors are from the Departments of Medicine and Pediatrics. The Chair of Medicine followed a very similar career path to mine and lived through some rather formative experiences at our institution that gave me incredible insight and helped me avoid mistakes. He was a great sounding board for my most challenging issues, including working with hospital administration and problematic faculty. The Chair of Pediatrics led the search committee that brought me to my chair position and was one of the major reasons I chose to come here. Both are what I'd call a "mensch" – a Yiddish term that is loosely translated as a "good person" but really means much more than that – to me, it stands for integrity and self-lessness, or the kind of person I'd want to be.

But whatever your stage of leadership, you'll find the mentorship from your peers to be invaluable. Those are the ones – often the only ones – who can truly relate to what you're going through and provide you with the insight you need to handle your most challenging situations. It's natural to feel sometimes like you're in competition with your peers, such as when competing over limited resources. However, it often becomes apparent (or at least it should!) that you will have more success by collaborating and aligning your goals rather than competing with each other.

After talking about the great mentorship I described above, I would be remiss not to describe the great joy and fulfillment you can obtain by providing mentorship to others. I found myself, after being chair for a couple of years, reaching out to new chairs to offer help and assistance however I could. But just like your relationship with your coach, the chemistry is important, and you have to be able to admit when you don't have it with the other person, despite best intentions. Plus, mentorship has nicely evolved over time from having a single mentor having a mentorship group, with the guiding principle that your mentors, however many you have, are committed to your development and success. Successful mentorship can be like a tapestry made up of multiple sources woven together, all providing a slightly different perspective that allows you to mature and develop.

Now that you've gained some insight into your character and personality as a leader, let's focus on your team and how to make it function as highly as possible, leading to success for everyone, including you.

Your Team

3

There would not be a leader without a team. So, unless you're a one-man/woman show, you're going to need an understanding of how to build a team. The focus should be on the end result(s), and people need to be on the same page as to what the goals are, so that they can concentrate on achieving them. In medicine, the goals are different based on the individual group; thus, establishing the vision and goals for your group is essential, so that they know the scope, steps, and potential obstacles. All too often, teams are left to make assumptions as to what the goals are; this leads to uncertainty, questioning, and a lack of faith or trust in you as a leader. Setting the goals, and reminding people of them periodically, will help keep your group oriented and focused.

Remember, *every* team has dynamics, and there is no such thing as a perfectly functional team. I like to think of it as constantly striving toward optimal functionality – every team has an optimal functional level, at least intuitively, and pretty much any team member can (or should) find resonance with that concept. After all, not many people enjoy being on a dysfunctional team. We often settle for it, but mostly because we don't take the necessary steps to make the team function better and just accept dysfunction as "the norm." This becomes exhausting and a bit defeatist. The teams that are willing to take growth steps toward better functionality not only are more likely to achieve their goals – they're also more likely to enjoy the process and sign up for more group projects in the future!

Who Is on Your Team: Did You Inherit It or Are You Assembling It?

When you assume a new leadership position, you may be inheriting a team that already exists or have to build one from scratch. Most teams are a combination of preexisting/established members and new people that you can bring in of your own choosing. Those members are very different, with some inherent dynamics that you need to be very conscious of as a leader.

You are not the first person to think of going on a "listening tour" when you start with your new team. But that is not to say that it is not a good idea – it is! However, *how* you listen is as important as the fact that you're going on the tour, and probably more important. The team members that have inherited you as their leader may be wary, excited, optimistic, pessimistic, or anywhere on the spectrum. You may or may not have been their first choice as the new leader. Regardless, you will buy yourself quite a lot of clout by listening to their perspectives, truly listening, so that they actually feel heard. That way, when you have to make difficult decisions that you know will be contrary to their views or wishes, it will be somewhat easier, as you can recognize their position in the process, showing that you heard them, and transparently explain why you chose to take things in a different direction. Everyone knows that it is the leader's prerogative to make difficult and sometimes unpopular decisions; they find the pill easier to swallow when they know that you've done your best to hear different perspectives and weigh the options as objectively as possible.

So, how do you run an effective listening tour? I would suggest some combination of group and one-on-one meetings, depending on the size of the group. Smaller overall group sizes make 1:1 meetings more doable, and this is most often the most productive way to get to know people and help them feel heard. But there is one caveat: some people are very uncomfortable in a 1:1 situation with a person in a position of authority, so it's best not to make such meetings mandatory, letting people off the hook if they choose not to meet with you, for whatever reason. But if they do choose this, at some point it will be important to understand why, as their behavior will likely impact the team regardless of the reason.

When in the 1:1 meetings, you can demonstrate your effective listening through several mechanisms. First, reduce distractions (anything that buzzes, beeps, or flashes) and make good eye contact. This shows that you truly care about what they have to say and that you don't want anything to distract you (or them). When I was a junior faculty, I vividly remember my meetings with my chair; they were always short, probably no more than 10–15 minutes, but I remember her eyes never wavered from mine, and I knew I had her complete and undivided attention. Sure, it was intimidating, but maybe that was because of her position of authority. But I had no doubt that she heard what I had to say and that I had a clear path forward after leaving her office.

Second, truly listen. What beliefs, values, or reasoning give greater perspective to their point of view? Ask for examples to better explain their position. Make sure you understand by summarizing and paraphrasing their comments, thus communicating a desire to really get what they are saying. Show sensitivity when appropriate to the emotional tone of what they are presenting. Remember, listening means not interrupting, or only interrupting when absolutely necessary. An interruption in a conversation implies that what you have to say is more important than *what they were already saying*. So use interruptions infrequently. Now, of course, there are caveats to this too, such as if you need to clarify something they're saying or have said, or if they're being repetitive, disorganized, or going off topic. The latter is more tricky. Few will mind being interrupted for clarification of what they're saying – that's a sign you were not only listening but that you truly wanted to understand. But some will ramble aimlessly, which has the double effect of making them feel disrespected when you have to cut them off and you tuning out due to a lack of pertinence in the conversation. So, as hard as it can be sometimes, redirecting the conversation may be a necessary part of your role as a leader, and over time people will understand your patterns of communication and the need to establish efficiency. Although some people are naturally garrulous, others only become so when they are nervous or excited, which is often the case when meeting with leadership. You can recognize this together, tell them it's okay and that you're truly listening, and you can both walk out of the room feeling good about the conversation. If you simply get frustrated and don't redirect them, the feeling for both parties at the end of the meeting may be quite different.

Third, take notes. It is perfectly fine to write things down or type into your computer as you're meeting, and you should inform the other person that that's what you're doing (and not something else, particularly if you're using a laptop and they can't see your screen). These notes will serve as points of reference, areas for clarification, and for a follow-up email or documentation to make sure you've heard each other correctly. This helps the other person to feel that not only were they heard but also their points were noted for current and future consideration. They will feel valued.

Finally, it's helpful to send a summary of the conversation, typically by email. Once again, this shows them that you've listened and that you've processed the information. It also gives them an opportunity to clarify any misunderstandings or misconceptions. It helps with goal setting and serves as a great reference point for future meetings. This may seem like a lot of work, and it certainly can be cumbersome. But it sends a great message to those you're leading, and in future meetings you can ask *them* to write up the summary and send it to you for review, completing the process in reverse.

Once you've gotten to know the members of the team you inherit, you can then bring on new people of your own choice. You will have a better idea of the existing culture, and maybe some of the strengths and weaknesses of existing team members, and can thus strategically hire to fill gaps in your team, augmenting strengths, compensating for weakness, and adding necessary diversity so that the group can grow together.

Assessing the Personalities and Strengths/Weaknesses of All Individuals

As you start to get to know your group, it's helpful to take note of personality characteristics, both constructive and challenging, that may impact the group dynamic and success. To be clear, this is not in an effort to be punitive or even necessarily change people, but more for you to be aware of people's tendencies and how they interact with you and the group. We all have personality traits, and we're all different from one another. Some of our traits are very helpful in the group dynamic, whereas others can be destructive. Awareness of yourself and others will go a long way in making you an effective leader.

There are a number of useful tools available to assess potential hires, or even to assess people you know will be on your team already due to their established position. At the time that the team is coming together under a new leader, it is a great opportunity for these types of assessments across the board. Not only does it provide you with awareness of their personality tendencies, but it also provides them with some self-awareness that emphasizes the importance of understanding one's own personality as it pertains to the team. The 16pf tool (www.16pf.com) and the Hogan Personality Inventory (www.hoganassessments.com) are two web-based tools that are relatively quick and simple personality assessments, and both have gone through years of study in the business world to help validate their utility.

Now, it is not as easy in most cases to know all of another person's personality traits, and usually only time will reveal someone's true character and tendencies. But it's perfectly acceptable as you're getting to know people on your team to ask them what they think they bring to the team and what areas they'd like to improve, both about the team and about themselves. Keep in mind that most people have not been asked this by their leaders, and also that most people like talking about themselves and can be quite revealing when put to the task of self-analysis. Some will "wear it on their sleeve" – everything is out in the open, what you see is what you get, and there isn't a lot of second-guessing as to where they stand. Others may be more reserved or reticent at first, and their true character only starts to show over time.

People may also behave differently in a one-on-one meeting with you compared with in a group, and the group dynamic can be truly fascinating! Although it's natural for the group leader to run the meeting and direct the conversation, it's very helpful to have moments of give and take between team members, where the leader sits back and observes. Although the meeting needs to run on time and work through an agenda, observing the group dynamic can be incredibly revealing over time, especially as they become more comfortable with you, and is a great way for you to better understand who is going to be most helpful to the group's success and why, as well as how to give helpful advice and instruction, both individually and to the group as a whole. It is less threatening when you give advice to an entire group at once, mixing words of encouragement with suggestions for how to more effectively communicate. But sometimes you'll have to have a private conversation with a team member whose efforts are detrimental to the group, often unintentionally. You'll need to have some common sense, especially early on, about when to have these private conversations versus public guidance to the group. When in doubt, err toward the former so as to not embarrass any single individual and terrify the rest of the group!

Keep in mind that, over time, the group will start to develop its own identity. Your role is to shape it, build the culture, and gently or firmly guide things in a positive, goal-oriented direction. You may need to nip at the edges to ensure a good group dynamic, but if you can groom a well-functioning team, you will be more likely to achieve goals and generate satisfaction for the team itself in doing so and personal fulfillment for yourself in the process.

The Importance of Diversity

Much has been said and written about the importance of diversity, equity, and inclusion in recent years, and hopefully it has become somewhat intuitive that diversity makes a group stronger. But it may be most useful to reframe your thinking about diversity as a tool rather than a goal. All too often, we end up thinking of diversity as a box that needs to be checked, as if once you have a certain composition to the group you've accomplished someone else's idea of a good thing. But this falls short of what great importance diversity can and should hold for your group.

Think about the roots of the word "diversity" – to diverge in some way. Diversity does not just mean a different representation in gender, race, culture, or preferences, but also a difference in viewpoint, which may be *because of* the person's gender, race, culture, or preferences, or for other reasons altogether. The beauty of diversifying your group is that you gain new and different perspectives that help you to better understand and solve problems, enabling the group to achieve its mutual goals. Remember, the goals of the group often remain independent of the group's composition, but the makeup of the group helps dictate how it views and approaches obstacles and processes, and the greater the diversity of the group, the higher its chances for success.

Diversity fails when people are closed-minded. In fact, one has to be open-minded in order to accept a viewpoint that is different from one's own, or one that challenges them in an uncomfortable way. Unless the group's goals are ridiculously simple and easily achieved, which is almost never the case, you'll likely encounter some conflict along the way, as you try to navigate through different perspectives. An important step for the group will be to embrace the conflict, not shy away from it, as the tension points are necessary nodes for the group to work through. Your job as leader is to help them navigate these channels so that they don't want to kill each other in the process!

As you work to increase the diversity of the group, you'll need to keep in mind two seemingly competing principles: (1) you want people with different viewpoints, so you can best explore all avenues to problem-solving, and (2) you want the group to have good chemistry. An often-quoted model is Abraham Lincoln's cabinet, the subject of Doris Kearns Goodwin's book, *Team of Rivals*. Although formed somewhat for political reasons, Lincoln's cabinet was comprised of very strong individuals with often vigorously competing opinions and viewpoints. This served him well in a very difficult time, and whether or not he catered to one or another viewpoint, his diverse group likely felt heard and respected for their opinions, even if a different course of action was taken. Now, of course, most of us don't have the innate leadership abilities of Abraham Lincoln, but neither do we typically face the abhorrent challenges he and his team faced in the 1860s. But we can learn from the principles of his team and how he managed it.

Another leadership book I've found particularly helpful is *Five Dysfunctions of a Team* by Patrick Lencioni. Through a long illustrative case, Lencioni eloquently outlines the hurdles overcome (or not) by a fictional business team. Leadership in the business world is very different from the medical field, but many of the same principles apply, and again, a diverse and strongly opinionated team is a good thing. Lencioni builds a conceptual pyramid for the reader, and at the base of the pyramid is TRUST between the team members, including the leader. This sounds conceptually easy: of course, you'd like to trust your team members. But he makes the point that very few teams actually establish the kind of *deeper trust* that is necessary to work together as a team. From the very first meetings, team members are feeling each other out, consciously or subconsciously noting personality traits and tendencies, mannerisms of speaking or communicating, and especially body language. The point is not to stop doing that – it is human and natural – but to move past the initial judgments and impressions and work toward a deeper trust of each other, recognizing the value of each team member in achieving the common goals of the group.

Which brings up an important concept to reiterate: the team needs frequent refocusing on the common goals and vision. If it feels like people are getting off track or too into the weeds, it's a good time to refocus the group on what your overall goals are, either for that meeting or for the group as a whole, whether it's a residency, division, department, or medical center. People need these refreshers in order to take a step back, recalibrate, and see how what they're bogged down in at that moment fits into the bigger picture. It's very easy to get lost in seemingly meaningful dead ends or small skirmishes; the leader can bring everyone back to the table, figuratively and literally, and reinforce the focus that all groups lose from time to time. It's natural and expected; the leader need not get frustrated with these moments but rather realize it's time to step in and bring the group back together. Or even just take a break!

The diversity of your group will be its greatest strength over time. If you can bring together dissimilar individuals with different perspectives who can rally around a common goal, you have the building blocks for a high-performing group. But along with the TRUST that your group will need to grow with each other (and you) over time, there's another quality that needs to be there from day one: RESPECT. Each group member needs to feel from the outset that they will be respected and valued for what they bring to the team, and that this respect will endure. The leader is the one who ensures that they garner and maintain that respect for one another. The respect for everyone from day one is only accomplished by some prework – establishing not only the goals for the group but also the principles for how they'll treat and interact with each other. This can be done *prior to* the first meeting of the group, or *during* the first meeting. Both can be effective.

If you feel that you have a valuable but potentially difficult team member, you can meet with them prior to the group meeting to set expectations and even to voice your concerns about behavior within the group. Conversely, if you have a valuable but potentially vulnerable team member, you can provide them with reassurance prior to the group meeting that you will stand by your principles of communication and respect, and that you will have their back in the group setting. I've also found it very important to reiterate your principles of respect and communication in the first group setting as well, even if some members have heard it before. As you're setting your vision for the group and learning about each other, you can discuss the "red lines" that are not to be crossed, such as any form of discrimination, harassment, or disrespect. That way, everyone has heard them, and they're starting on an equal playing field. And then you send it out in the minutes so you can refer back to it when needed! (And it often *is* needed down the road . . .)

Now you're ready to bring your diverse group to the table, set some goals, agree to some crucial concepts, and get to know each other better, so that they can be a truly functional group. In Chapter 6, we'll get into how you run an effective meeting with the group. But now let's dive into the potential layers within your group.

Establishing Midlevel Leadership (If Appropriate)

Depending on the size of your group, you may need to develop layers of leadership. What I will describe here will be most relevant at the departmental level, but hopefully some of the concepts will be applicable to levels above and below that.

You may find that your group has grown to a critical mass, and you're discovering that connections and communications are becoming unwieldy, or just that you're not able to have as effective a relationship with all group members. It does not mean that you're less effective as a leader, but it's very time-consuming to connect frequently and effectively with everyone in a large group, and sometimes you need layers. This also allows you to give leadership opportunities to others, which many in medicine are looking for and appreciate. And then comes the great joy and fulfillment of mentoring them as leaders as well and seeing them rise and succeed! You can still maintain a connection, a meaningful one, with the larger group as a whole, and hopefully over time they see you working as a unit with the midlevel leadership.

To be more concrete, the leadership structure in an academic department can be made up of multiple layers of leadership. Right below you as the chair/chief, you can have any number of vice chairs, but keep in mind that the more vice chairs you have, the more diluted their leadership feels and becomes. In my first experience as vice chair, I was the "clinical" vice chair, in charge of everything within the clinical realm, which included educational efforts within the department. It was an unbelievably arduous job, but also very gratifying! The chair and I were very clear about who was responsible for what, but also that I reported to him and that he had the ultimate say in our "joint" decision-making. This clear delineation of duties created a great and satisfying working relationship, but also required a tremendous amount of work on my part.

When I became chair myself at a different institution, I took my time before assigning my first vice chair, a translational researcher, who became a research vice chair to complement my strengths as more of a clinical researcher and educator. This was a very necessary position to hire into, as I certainly did not have the bandwidth to build up both the clinical and educational programs as well as developing translational and basic science within the department. We now also have clinical and educational vice chairs, which complement each other well, and we maintain clear lines of responsibility and reporting. I've seen vice chair models ranging from one to eight people; there is no right or wrong number, but rather the number should be dictated by the needs and missions of the department. For example, a very research-heavy department might have a vice chair for clinical research and another for translational/basic science research. Some very large departments might also benefit from an "executive vice chair" that oversees the other vice chairs. But then you have to ask what the role of the chair is and how it is distinct from the executive vice chair. In still another model, most useful when an institution has multiple affiliated sites, having such titles as "chief," "chair," or "vice chair" at the sites apart from the mothership are all reasonable. Again, as long as everyone understands their role and responsibilities, it can work well.

Another layer below the vice chairs could include your division chiefs, inpatient and outpatient medical directors, and educational leadership (residency program and medical school clerkship directors). Depending on what kind of department you have, you could have anywhere from three to ten such positions. For example, within Internal Medicine, you would have division chiefs for cardiology, pulmonary/critical care, renal, and so on; within Surgery, you might have division chiefs for colorectal surgery, urologic surgery, cardiothoracic surgery, and so on. Each of these divisions might be comprised of anywhere from one to ten or more members. You might think that having a division chief for a division comprised of one person sounds ridiculous, but it can be very useful for (1) giving that person the representation they might not otherwise get, (2) earmarking future growth of that division that you think is likely or important, and (3) grooming another future leader within your department, provided you think that person has leadership potential and wants to lead.

For a lack of a better term, I'll describe this group of division chiefs, medical directors, and educational leaders as "midlevel leadership." This is an extremely important group in any department, and all too often there is little guidance and focus for this group, and they fail to benefit from learning from each other. They're highly intertwined, frequently impacting each other in ways that may not always be obvious or intuitive until brought to the surface. All too often, the leaders in this group will see themselves as masters of their own domain, always on the lookout for their constituents and their interests. This is, of course, laudable, but they will be more effective (including for their constituents!) when they realize how they fit into the larger puzzle of the department. Rather than having them feel like they're competing for limited resources, it is better to help them understand how they fit into the overall mission, and how they can contribute to the greater success of the department that will help all boats to rise, including theirs.

In our department, we went through an interesting, deliberate exercise. I asked all of the midlevel leadership to write down what they thought made a good division chief, medical director, or educational leader. I asked for this to be either high level or fine detail, whatever they wanted and thought was important. I then collated the concepts (except for those that were truly esoteric and impertinent to the larger group), and we discussed them as a group, eventually categorizing them and listing them in order of importance. This took multiple sessions of vetting and discussion. I then said I'd like for us to have a "leadership charter" that we could all agree to. I reminded them that this was not me dictating to them what their roles and responsibilities were, it was *their* concepts of what a good leader in their positions should provide for their group. Funnily, the group then realized that their laundry list of leadership qualities and concepts was a bit intimidating and long! This was an "ah hah" moment for our group, when they got perhaps their first or most dramatic insight into what it means and requires to be an effective leader in medicine. It was daunting and intimidating but also exciting and invigorating.

Once we finalized the document (with the understanding that it was a "living" document that could be amended in the future), I asked the group to sign the charter. I know, this sounds a bit ridiculous – it's not as if we were signing the Declaration of Independence. But symbolically, it *was* like that, or perhaps our "Declaration of Inter-Dependence." We had created this conceptual document together, vetted it, agreed to it, and now we would stand by it. It was perhaps one of the most profound moments of my career in medicine to see each person take up the pen, one by one, and sign.

From that point forward, our group was *together*. We had aligned our goals and agreed to common qualities and characteristics that we envisioned being effective for the department. Shortly thereafter, the COVID-19 pandemic struck (see Chapter 9, "Leadership in a Crisis"), but all of our prework served us well, and we were able to handle this extreme adversity better as a group. We had an understanding of each other's roles and how each group fit into the overall mission of the department. We had established trust in one another in the process, a kind of trust that can only develop through working together on a project. Working on the project of what makes a good leader is an easy and fun project; working on how to handle a pandemic as a department is much harder. Both can make the group stronger, if navigated well.

Let's now discuss how to mentor all of these different leaders in your group.

Establishing Mentorship across All Levels

Mentorship means different things to different people. In medicine, people classically equate mentorship with research guidance, and although this clearly still exists and is extremely important, there are other types of mentorship that can be particularly beneficial in the medical community, including educational mentorship, clinical mentorship, psychological mentorship, "life" mentorship, and leadership mentorship. Although here I will concentrate on the last of these, they may all come into play, depending on the phenotype of the leader you're mentoring.

The first steps in establishing the mentor–mentee relationship are to set the expectations regarding each other's roles, the frequency and structure of meetings, and how to crisis manage and problem solve together. It helps if each sees themselves as an enabler – you enabling the success of the leader under you, and them enabling the success of those they are leading. You thus establish a mutual goal, the overall success of the group(s) that you both are responsible for, either directly or indirectly. For example, let's use a vice chair (VC) of education, mentoring a residency program director (PD). The PD may be responsible for not just the residents but also the assistant PD(s) and the residency program coordinator as well. The VC can help the PD understand their leadership structure and serve as a sounding board for residency issues (including how to help counsel problematic residents), as well as planning for new educational initiatives within the residency. The VC can also talk with the PD about their personal style, including communication, leadership, or teaching, and what strengths and weaknesses they bring to all of these domains. It's a great relationship for looking at 360s as well, helping to process the results and come up with action plans as to how to improve, or at least be aware of potential trends or shortcomings.

Periodic meetings between the mentor and mentee are essential; the frequency can be dictated by need – how much is going on in a given section or domain at a given time – or simply for the sake of regularity, maintaining the importance of the relationship over time. The meetings should include an agenda, and this can come either from the mentor or mentee, but typically the latter. Make sure the appropriate amount of time is allotted, typically 30–60 minutes, depending on the number and nature of issues. The "trap" of these meetings is that they can turn into boring updates, such as on recent publications or talks, which, although nice and somewhat important, are more for pleasing a mother/father figure. More effective meetings center around problem-solving, often using specific examples or instances, HR discussions (of which there is a seemingly endless stream, regardless of where you work!), and sometimes more enjoyable planning or strategizing for the group, where innovation comes to the fore and you can be creative. These moments are often when the mentor and mentee feel that they're getting the most out of the relationship, building respect for what each brings to the table.

Although it's tempting to use your meetings as periodic check-ins, this can lead to a stale mentor–mentee relationship over time. Of course, sometimes there are no major issues to discuss, but do not be afraid to tackle bigger, thorny issues if you see them. This takes your mentor–mentee relationship from ordinary to productive, meaningful, and impactful. Neither one of you will feel that you're wasting time, and your trust in each other will only grow. However, if discussing the more difficult issues is not working, leading to tension or discomfort, you need to take a step back and understand why. Is the person defensive and not able to receive feedback well? Is there something in your delivery that is rubbing the other person the wrong way? Is there another factor that neither one of you are considering, or some "skeleton in the closet" that is trying to poke its skull out? Go back to basics – why are you there together? What are you trying to accomplish? What are your mutual goals? You are there to help – mentorship is all about helping and finding the most effective ways to be helpful based on your needs and personality traits.

How you end the meetings is as important as how you begin them. Look back over your agenda – did you get to everything on it? Did you address each topic satisfactorily? Is there homework? Recap the meeting, both in person and preferably by email as well, so that you both leave on the same page as to action plans, homework, and follow-up. This serves as a great reference point and is a useful reminder of what was said at the time, given that both of you likely have very busy lives and can't remember everything! Spending an extra five minutes at the end to type up a summary is like gold for future meetings and ends up saving both of you a lot of future frustration and wheel spinning.

Mentorship is not one-size-fits-all, nor is it a good idea to put all your eggs in one mentorship basket. It's not like finding your soulmate; you can, and should, have more than one mentor, and you should encourage your mentees to have other mentors as well. And this mentorship group should be diverse too, providing a wide array of perspectives and thinking processes that will help the individual to see their issues from multiple angles. Be humble enough to know that your mentee may get better advice on a given issue from someone other than you. Embrace those moments, learn from them, and even celebrate them. As the mentee sees your acceptance and growth from this different perspective, their admiration and respect for you will likely only increase. Again, it is about the mentee feeling that you have their best interests in mind, whether the solutions come from you or someone else. Think of mentorship as "by committee," including for yourself. As a chair, I look for mentorship wherever I can find it – from other chairs, my hospital chief medical officer and CEO, my dean, and even from chairs in other institutions. The more sounding boards you have, the more perspective you gain, making your decisions better informed, either consciously or subconsciously.

Lastly, it is important to understand the difference between "mentorship" and "sponsorship." I refer the reader to the excellent article by Ayyala et al., (Mentorship is not enough) but briefly, sponsorship is focused on specific career opportunities, such as serving on national committees or review boards, leading a clinical trial, or presenting at a national conference. Sponsorship is particularly important for people or groups that commonly are disadvantaged for such specific opportunities, usually underrepresented groups such as women and people of color. It is a way to advocate proactively for people you are leading, so that they can get coveted career opportunities and advance their professional goals. As you're working with your mentee, you can actively discuss what opportunities for which they would like your help in terms of sponsorship. It is one thing to forward them an email from a national society with a "Call for Abstracts"; it is quite another to sponsor them to put on a course at a national congress or to serve on a national committee within their area of interest, or to nominate them to serve as the site principal investigator for a clinical trial at your institution. Given your position of leadership, you are best able to advocate within your circles for career-advancing opportunities for your mentees. This process should be deliberate, proactive, and overt.

Recruiting and Retaining

One of the most important skill sets for a leader, especially one responsible for hiring and building, is recruiting and retaining. Bringing in good team members does not happen by itself – it takes hard work, patience, and a strong ego for when you get turned down by a potential recruit or when you're unable to retain a person you want to keep. There is no magic formula for how to recruit the best people for your group, but there are several principles that may be helpful for you.

First and foremost, make sure that you and the recruit are on the same page about the position you're recruiting for. You might advertise that you're recruiting a new division chief for trauma surgery, but the trauma group might be small (1–3 people) or huge (15–20 people), and the administrative duties may vary widely, as will the personalities and skill sets needed. Not all jobs are created equal, and it's best for both sides to come in with a clear understanding of the tasks at hand and the expectations, as well as the timeline.

Second, elaborate on the culture and mission of the institution overall, so that the recruit has a sense of what the priorities are, as well as the culture and type of people who tend to come there and find fulfillment. For example, someone with a heavy research portfolio might not be satisfied or fit in at a place where clinical care and education are the major emphases; alternatively, they might be the perfect recruit if the institution (or you) was trying to build in a different direction, such as growing the research enterprise. It's all a matter of timing and fit.

Third, for all you Clint Eastwood fans out there, I like to be upfront about "the good, the bad, and the ugly." I deliberately tell them what is imperfect about the place or the position and what would be needed to accommodate or fix things if they were to take the job. All too often, people are sold a lemon and question the integrity of the person who recruited them ("You never told me about that!"). No one wants to be sold a lemon or find out that their job was a lemon after the fact. Be proactive about letting them know, by standing in their shoes, what you'd be concerned about if you were to take the job yourself. Your credibility will go through the roof with this, and you'll likely get a person who truly understands the position, warts and all, and is ready to roll up their sleeves and get to work. Worst-case scenario, they are turned off by the job and decide not to come. But that's for the best as well, as neither of you will have wasted time in a situation doomed to fail.

Fourth, "show the love." People naturally want to feel wanted and appreciated, especially if they're looking for a change. It is perfectly okay to try to recruit someone who may not have been looking for a new job – in fact, they'll likely find it very flattering that someone has gone out of their way to recognize their talents. But the love does not stop there; frequent, honest, and direct communication makes the recruit feel highly valued, in essence grooming them for the position.

Fifth, don't settle. Sometimes it's enticing to try to seal the deal with someone who is "close enough" or who you think you can "coach up" to the position. Sometimes you don't have a choice because of time or other pressures, but usually you can take your time and find the best fit for the job. A's beget more A's, and B's beget more B's (or C's). Don't be seduced by the CV – if they're not a good fit for your program, they'll declare themselves sooner or later. Your track record in recruiting good people will lay the foundation for many years to come.

Sixth, consider having a standing interview committee, comprised of you and some leaders who understand the basic principles of good interviewing and vetting of candidates and who are able to give you honest and direct input. Depending on the position, you may have ad hoc members of the interview committee, and they will need to be coached to the successful principles of interviewing, but your core group will give you the most mileage. It is also helpful to establish standardized interview questions to cover multiple important domains, asked by the same interviewer in the same way to each candidate. This creates an even playing field for all candidates, which they typically appreciate.

Finally, *always* vet the candidate thoroughly – not just with the references the candidate provides, but also from other people they work with. It is easy to get lazy toward the end of a recruitment and not feel compelled to take this extra step, or perhaps be reluctant for anything to derail the process so close to the end, but this is one mistake that will come back to bite you if you're not diligent. You might get sold a "lemon" anyway, but it won't be for lack of due diligence.

Retaining good people is as important as recruiting them. In fact, it may be even more painful to lose someone in whom you've invested a lot of time and energy, and who is a productive and valued team member. People will commonly leave to pursue better opportunities, but don't let the loss occur from a lack of appreciation on your part. Keep your eyes open and ears perked for signs of discontent and restlessness, and be proactive about trying to ensure a valuable team member's sense of happiness and fulfillment. This can be done through addressing whatever is making them less than satisfied, or by sitting down with them and mapping out their next steps and future career should they stay. Remember, the process of recruiting is time-consuming and often painful, with many unknowns and risks. It is often far better to retain a good team member than to recruit and groom a replacement.

Operating Principles

Once you've assembled your team, you have to be very clear about roles and responsibilities. Without overt delineation of who is responsible for what, team members will inevitably step on each other's toes, fail to work together, or worse, fail to take responsibility at all. One of the most useful tools is a "RACI" matrix (responsibility assignment matrix) – this makes it clear who is *Responsible* for specific tasks, who will be held *Accountable* for a task's successful completion, who needs to be *Consulted*, and who needs to be *Informed*. This centers the focus of a group on individual tasks and what their exact role is, taking out the guesswork. Those *Responsible* for a given task will work either singly or as a small group to do the actual work. Usually one person is *Accountable* for overseeing the work and is the problem solver or leader of the task force. They report up and down, overseeing the task group and reporting to the overall leader of the group. *Consulted* persons provide input to the work in progress, helping guide the process, and are active participants. *Informed* people are typically group leaders or primary stake-holders (such as a board of directors), who have a stake in the project and its outcome but are not directly involved and do not provide formal consultation.

Another important concept is decision rights – who gets to make deci-sions? Is it only the leader, or are there group decisions, or some mix of the two? There are benefits and drawbacks to both decision-making structures, and it's helpful to be overt about how decisions will be made for a given situation. You may find it's best to have the group leader make the "hard" decisions, taking on the sole burden/blame of the outcome of the decision. Alternatively, the group may be more engaged if they understand they'll have a say/vote in the hard decisions. They may feel that this gives them more of a stake in the process, leading to more ownership and growth. Depending on your style and your group, you may choose one or the other approach. But whichever you choose, your group will function better if you are overt about it from the get-go.

Now that you've formed your team and established some lines of communication, let's turn next to establishing your vision for the group.

Setting the Vision

At once daunting and exciting, your vision statement for your group, presented both orally and in writing, is one of your most important and memorable acts as a leader. It should be given a great deal of advance thought and planning, and you should be sure to vet it with a number of people who will give you good and frank advice. Although they can be intimidating, vision statements are usually full of positivity and forward-thinking, are a great source of inspiration to your group, and serve as the ultimate frame of reference. In other words, you're unlikely to fail with this, but most statements will end up being ordinary. But it is an opportunity to be *extra*ordinary, for you to set the tone for your group as their leader. An opportunity not to be wasted.

Mission versus Vision

Although often conflated, the mission and vision statements are two different things. The mission statement should be very brief, usually no more than a sentence or two. It is high level and speaks to the core principles that guide the group, the key objective(s). It should incorporate concepts that everyone can agree to, serving as a rallying cry. It should not be controversial but rather inspiring, easy to grasp and agree to, and unifying for the group. You may refer to your mission statement frequently, especially in times of strife, so it's best to get thoughtful input and buy-in from the group ... which leads to another common mistake: most leaders think they need to come up with the mission statement all by themselves. It is healthier to think of your role as creating the first draft, remaining open to suggestion and revision by the group. In fact, that's *how* you'll get the most buy-in for the present and future, with the whole group taking ownership of their guiding principles. The mission statement should optimally be a joint endeavor, etched in a soft stone if you will, malleable enough to be revisited and amended in the future. But rarely should mission statements require a major overhaul, unless the overall goals of the group change drastically, which is rare in medicine.

Another concept of major importance to your mission statement is that it should be consistent and align with the overarching missions above it, such as those of the department, the institution, the medical school, and the university. If you see your mission in isolation, you are likely to run afoul of some of the missions of these higher entities, potentially putting the goals of your group at risk. Before drafting your mission statement for your group, consider rereading the mission statements for the groups above you. The more you can align goals and principles, the more successful your group will be; this is because it's more likely that your goals will be mutually beneficial with the institution overall. The details of your vision statement can be more specific to your group, but the mission statement should be closely aligned with at least the nearest governing body above you.

I have included a sample mission statement in Appendix 1, specific to our neurology department as of 2021. Let's turn next to the vision statement, which is far more complex and detailed.

Vision Statement: Addressing All of the Pillars

The vision statement will naturally be longer and much more detailed than the mission statement, but it should also remain succinct and have resonance. The structure and organization are important, touching on the central themes of your group with a clear and practical voice that is easy to understand. Also important, but often overlooked, are metrics associated with the central themes. These can either be integrated into your themes as you discuss them or separated out in a different section. An example from our department is in Appendix 1, where we chose to separate out the metrics. Overall, your vision statement should be no more than two pages, optimally a single page.

And now let's consciously change the word I've been using, "themes," to the word "pillars." This may sound lofty and grandiose, but remember, these are the bedrock for your group, what they're going to refer back to for months and maybe years to come. So, they are indeed important and deserving of the name "pillars." You may choose to have anywhere from three to five pillars for your group; there is no magic number, but rather the number is dictated by the goals and aims of your group. The classic pillars for most groups in medicine, at least academic medicine, are Clinical, Education, and Research. In our department, we added two more, Administration and Culture, consciously elevating their importance so that the entire group could focus on their relevance to the overall mission of the department. Remember, your vision statement will always reflect back on your mission statement; the two should be in perfect harmony.

Whatever pillars you choose, it is essential to make the goals specific. For example, for our Research pillar, we specified the importance of clinical, translational, and basic science research, and then outlined such metrics as highly impactful publications in well-respected journals, leading impactful investigator-initiated studies, providing research support and mentorship to junior faculty and trainees, attaining National Institutes of Health (NIH) and extramural funding, and the importance of cross-disciplinary collaboration, among others. For the Education pillar, metrics became more tricky, but we eventually focused on the importance of teaching evaluations compared with local and national benchmarks, evidence of innovation in education (e.g. development of new courses or educational tools), quality publication in medical education research, resident surveys, Continuing Medical Education (CME) courses, and educational awards, both local and national.

The Clinical pillar is easy to rally around; no medical group has a problem conceptually with striving for clinical excellence. But what metrics apply to clinical excellence? This is less obvious. For an academic medical center, or even for the individual practicing clinician, one meaningful marker is being sent the most difficult and challenging cases, given your reputation and expertise in the field. But that's not easy to track. One can look at referrals in versus referrals out for specialized treatment, or perhaps patient satisfaction surveys compared with regional and national benchmarks, but these can be subjective or biased by factors outside of your control (e.g. if you treat a skewed population of mostly privileged patients versus underprivileged or non-English-speaking, or even if you live in one particular region versus another). Perhaps you can measure innovation in your care or diagnosis of patients, especially that emulated by others. I have always found "Best Doctors" lists to be highly subjective, and their methods opaque and unmeaningful, but they are available and used by some. Finally, perhaps the most objective and meaningful clinical metric is tracking outcomes for your patients by their disease state, compared with national benchmarks, adjusted for age, race, gender, socioeconomic status, and other important variables.

Regarding the two additional pillars, Administrative and Culture, you may or may not choose to include these in your vision statement. Or you may choose to present them in oral form only, not elevating them to the status of the written statement. But the Culture pillar is particularly important to most groups and having some overt conversation about it is helpful. Do you define your culture from within? Or do you look for external measures of your culture, or at least your culture's effect, from outside your group/department? Culture, or at least reputation, factors into national rankings, such as those run by Doximity and US News and World Report; actually, the reputation and ratings from peers factor more prominently than one might think. But these are rather crude tools. Other, perhaps more meaningful metrics might be performing wellness surveys to measure the effect of programs focused on wellness/burnout. Your efforts on diversity are crucial here as well, helping to define your culture as equitable, welcoming, and antiracist. Is your group seen as working together, or is it a collection of individuals doing their own thing? Does your group feel free from any form of discrimination or harassment, or do people feel like they have to watch their backs? I've certainly worked in both environments. One might say that the more high-powered environments naturally have some internal backstabbing . . . some might even say that some elbowing is good, that the competition drives them to excellence. But I'm not in that camp. I think you can achieve excellence *and* have a supportive culture that embraces equity, inclusion, and diversity.

Now that you've established your pillars and written them down, let's talk about how you present them. The written word is the bedrock, what you'll refer to in times of strife or reflection. But your oral presentation is an important opportunity for you to put passion and feeling into the words and may be remembered by your group for its inspiration (or lack thereof).

Getting Personal: Have Them See You as Human

Let's separate the "vision meeting" into (1) the first vision and (2) subsequent updates/resets (discussed at the end of this chapter, "Resetting the Vision Periodically"). Depending on your personality, you may find this anywhere from exciting to perfunctory, from daunting to advantageous. It may be helpful to hear that your group really *is* interested in hearing from you, as their leader, and that this meeting is different from most of your other meetings of the year. True, you won't resonate with everyone in the room every time, as they may not all come with the right mindset. But you can't control that, and usually the majority of your group is genuinely looking forward to hearing your vision and understanding a bit about what makes you tick as a leader. Of course, there are many approaches to how you hold your first meeting; what I describe below goes over some general principles, which, like anything in this book, you can choose to incorporate or ignore as you see fit!

Both the setting and time are important. You will want an engaged audience, free from distractions, both external and internal. Hold the meeting in a quiet room with enough chairs for everyone. Consider the layout of the room – I always prefer a round-table setup, where we're talking with each other, rather than one person at the head of the room with everyone else facing that person, which sets up a "talking at" scenario. The other distraction to eliminate is time pressures – if there is an important meeting, clinic, or surgery right after your vision talk, people may be distracted or concerned that your talk will go on too long or keep them from that next important task. So, set the expectations early – if you have an hour scheduled, consider taking only 30–45 minutes, leaving time for Q&A at the end. You can also let people know, at the end of that 30–45 minutes, that it's okay for them to leave if they have to (few will, out of respect for you and the stature of the meeting), as that helps relax the room and takes some pressure off. Now you're ready to begin.

Although it may be uncomfortable for you to talk about yourself, this is one instance in which you absolutely should – they actually do want to hear about you, how you got to this point, what principles are important to you, and what inspires you. Before you get to what you expect from the group, you can get personal – they want to know your story, as it not only tells them what motivates you but shows them a career path that they may want to emulate or learn from. Although this may not be your style, I find that sharing more "human" qualities about oneself can resonate with the group. For example, my father was a great man and also the leader of his neurology department. He was certainly a great inspiration to me and my career, but it was also important for the group to understand that I wasn't interested in being a leader just because my father had been one, and that I distinguished myself from him in various ways and styles, which helped them to see me as distinct from my greatest role model and truly invested in them for the right reasons. I spoke at length about my many failures and obstacles I had to overcome; I think this was helpful for them to see me as not of some "Ivy League" pedigree who was going to boss them around and tell them how things were going to be done under the new leadership. I also emphasized the importance of this being *our* group, *our* department, not mine. I was nominally the leader, but we all needed to take responsibility for the success of the department and of each other. I emphasized that the vast majority of people "clock in, clock out" of their daily jobs, often failing to get satisfaction or enjoyment from their work. I think this is a huge miss, especially in medicine, where there are so many opportunities to make a deep and meaningful difference in people's lives; medicine, perhaps unlike most fields, is rife with opportunities for fulfillment and joy. The naysayers will default to the glory days, when there wasn't so much paperwork or bureaucracy. But that's a cop-out, in my opinion. Medicine still, perhaps now more than ever, is a fantastic career and can be incredibly rewarding.

Your enthusiasm and passion, both for your position and for the group, needs to come through. Even if you're not a naturally effusive person, at least take the time to have them understand what this group means to you and why you're excited to lead it. You can go over your pillars, in as much details as you'd like, but remember to watch their body language to know that your message is resonating with your audience, that they can agree (at least in principle) to the goals you're setting, and that they have some initial trust, or perhaps "faith" is a better word, in you as a leader.

Setting Goals and Milestones as well as Timelines

Along with establishing metrics for your vision, it's helpful to your team to establish milestones and timelines. Like children that play better when they know the rules of the sandbox, adults in medicine, regardless of the stage, perform better when they have clear expectations of what they and the group are expected to achieve and when.

To accomplish this, you can work from your loftier, more abstract principles to concrete goals, some of which may be short term, others long term. Both are helpful. What are they expected to accomplish this year, versus three or five years down the road? As an example, we'd like to establish a comprehensive, multidisciplinary pain center, capitalizing on our strength in interventional pain, as well as the clinical and research opportunities for our population with the major public health problem, opioid addiction. Optimally, this would be a freestanding clinic, with a bustling outpatient provider practice incorporating neurology, rehabilitation medicine, psychiatry, and neurosurgery, with a complementary physical and occupational therapy suite and even a fluoroscopy suite for on-site outpatient procedures. Not only would this bring a high-quality clinical service for our patients, but it would also serve as a great educational opportunity for trainees and students (including a pain fellowship program) and a research opportunity tied to clinical innovations and studies, and would hopefully generate revenue for the department and medical center through professional and technical revenue. This dream is clearly not going to happen overnight, maybe not even in the first year. But you plant the seeds and start the process with the vision statement. Maybe in the first year you hire key faculty and start the application process for the fellowship program. Maybe in the second year you expand your clinical footprint to the point that you can develop a compelling business plan for the hospital administration, which can start thinking about fronting the capital to grow a center. In the three-to-five-year period, you start to see your vision grow to fruition.

Depending on the size and variety of the group(s) that you're leading, you can do this on several fronts. And as always, work with the group to help them develop their own vision (with your guidance), rather than telling them what their vision and goals should be. Thereby you create buy-in and ownership of the programs, and your group feels empowered to work together to achieve the commonly agreed-upon goals. The buy-in must start from day one: everyone performs best when they understand what the group is striving for and what their specific role is in the process.

Having Your Group Understand and Rally Behind Your Vision

Let's go back to your first vision statement and discussion. Your group needs to rally behind your vision or, better stated, your mutual vision, and to do so they need to have a good understanding of the vision. The vision is for the future of the group, not your future personally; you are there to facilitate and lead the group. So, when you discuss the vision at the first meeting, again, spend only half or at most three-fourths of the time presenting the vision and leave the remainder for questions and discussion. Depending on the group, you may or may not get much interaction at this stage, but even if they are quiet, at least they know they were given the opportunity to respond and question, rather than walking away with the impression that their opinion was not valued because you left no time to hear it.

After presenting the vision in person, send it out in written (electronic) form, and ask for comments/suggestions/edits. Again, you may not get much, but people will feel like they were part of the process, that their opinion mattered. Once you've assimilated all of the feedback, send out the final version of the vision statement (and call it "final" so they understand this is what was agreed to at that stage in the group's development) to the whole group, so that you all have it on record and can refer back to it as needed. People may never look at it, but they can if they need to. And that's the point – it's a reference to what was agreed to at a point in time, the bedrock for your group.

One last thing about your vision statement: be explicit about the "red lines" for the group (and for you as their leader). In our department, we made it very clear that we would not tolerate any form of discrimination or harassment, regardless of the basis, whether it be on gender, race, ethnicity, sexual orientation/preference, or anything else. This is not controversial; everyone can agree to it in the moment, and there is never any argument. But I promise you, discrimination, harassment, or maltreatment may come up at some point, and having this point of reference, both in written and oral forms, will serve you well if you do need to pursue disciplinary action. They cannot come back and say you were not clear on this issue – it's right there in black and white.

Resetting the Vision Periodically

Finally, remember that your vision statement is a "living" document – it should be revisited, typically on a yearly basis, with adjustments made by the group as needed. Most years, the adjustments will be minor, tweaking some specific priorities or metrics for part of the department. Some years, the changes will be more drastic and deliberate. For example, your group, division, or department may develop financial issues, necessitating an adjustment in practices, cost cutting, and maybe even furloughing some staff. In 2020, we faced the mutual crises of the COVID-19 pandemic and the Black Lives Matter (BLM) movement, both of which were particularly poignant for our institution, because we are a safety-net hospital serving a predominantly nonwhite population, and our patients were particularly hard hit by the pandemic, both medically and financially. We were very deliberate in our approaches to both the pandemic (see Chapter 9) and the BLM movement and recalibrated our vision for the department to reflect these changes. The vision statement served as the reference point for what we learned through experience and helped grow the identity of the group and solidify our bond with the overall mission of the institution ("Exceptional Care without Exception"). In a period of tremendous hardship, our department came together and rededicated itself to clinical care, education, and impactful research, including work specific to the pandemic as well as in the realms of social disparities and antiracism.

Let's talk next about how we built and grew this culture, as well as how to handle adversity and challenges to the culture, which are inevitable.

Building the Culture

We all toss around the word "culture" when we refer to our group or another, but what do we really mean by it? For me, culture means several things when referring to a group: identity, values, goals, principles. It also means the emotions that people feel as they come to work. I like to think of a positive culture as the feeling of excitement while walking or driving into work, the joy that they get when seeing their colleagues, the genuine smiles they show each other. Culture can also be defined from the outside – how is your group viewed by others, either at your institution or outside? Is your group viewed as "functional," in which the members get along with each other, work as a team, and accomplish important goals? Or does it carry a reputation of being a "difficult place to work"? Usually a culture is a mix of hardworking and driven, supporting and nurturing.

Few leaders are explicit about the culture of their group, but one can accomplish a great deal by having open and honest conversations about culture, asking questions like "Who are we now?" and "Who do we want to be?" The culture of your group may already be quite good, even on autopilot, but this does not mean you should not be overt and deliberate about how you talk about and recognize your culture, and how to avoid the possibility of deterioration due to a lack of maintenance. But most groups are not on autopilot and need to take necessary steps to establish who they want to be, as well as who they don't.

The focus of this chapter will be on building the culture of your group, navigating negative culture events, and maintaining and cultivating a positive culture that will endure over time.

Elements of Your Core Identity as a Group

As you begin to bring your group together, starting with the first meeting you can introduce the conversation of not only what the group wants to accomplish, but how they want to do it, together. And that "together" refers to the group's identity – what principles do they embrace when they work with each other, what do they value, what do they tolerate? This is not to say that every group will become some symbiotic, utopian entity in which everything always runs smoothly. That does not exist. Each group will have its unique dynamics, based on the unique individuals who comprise it. A group is raw material, but with preconceptions. You, as the leader, are responsible for helping them find their identity as a group.

But how is this typically done? The first meeting of the group usually starts with introducing the members, assuming everyone doesn't already know each other. But even introductions can be guided – in addition to giving their name, they could give what department/group they represent, what their position is within that group, why they think they were chosen to be part of your group, if applicable. Then you could ask them what they hope to get out of this new group – an unusual and maybe uncomfortable question for some, but it is also disarming and helps to get people on the right page or outline misconceptions or knowledge gaps. A surprising number of people may have little to no idea why they're part of your group or what is expected of them. I sometimes like to ask people to answer the question, "What makes you tick?" It's rather open-ended and can be answered in a number of ways. It may be best for you as the leader to be the first to answer the question, so that others have a good example to follow, and they know what you mean. Rather than just boringly going around the room in a circle having people say their names, you can start the meeting with some meat and substance without losing anyone off the bat. And you certainly won't lose people's interest!

I like to be explicit in establishing core values for the group – who do we want to be, not just what do we want to accomplish. Certainly the goals are highly important, establishing what they're striving for, making them goal-oriented. But *how* they get there by working together is less commonly discussed and is what will separate your group from a bad group or even a good group, helping it to become a *great* group. So the first core value I like to emphasize is the value of effective communication. Effective communication allows for a healthy, diverse discussion, all the while maintaining decorum and respect. This is not to say that the conversation should be devoid of humor – humor is incredibly effective and helpful to a group. But humor needs to be used wisely and respectfully, never making any individual or part of the group feel marginalized or denigrated. One of my biggest pet peeves is interruptions in conversations. If Tom interrupts Mary midsentence, it can send the message that what he has to say is more important than what Mary *was already saying*, to the point that he felt empowered to shut her down. Some call this "mansplaining" when a man does it to a woman, but it can feel demeaning regardless of the people involved (although more so when there are gender or racial differences). Respectful discourse is a core value, and communication and respect go hand in hand. (Now, if Mary is inappropriately loquacious and is detrimental to the group on that basis, that's another issue, and a place for you to step in as the leader to help guide the conversation, maybe having a private conversation with Mary about her respect for others by letting them have a chance to talk too.)

On the other hand, if the conversation is too militaristic, it can become stifling, and you don't get the diverse representation, creativity, and fleshing out of ideas that you need. Respectful communication and lively discourse are not mutually exclusive and can peacefully coexist. As your group develops trust in one another, with you stepping in to guide the conversation when needed, their comfort level grows and they feel more at ease sharing their ideas, even their more daring or controversial ideas, all the while maintaining respect for the rest of the group. You, as the leader, may find yourself being a bit heavy-handed in the first few meetings, guiding a healthy conversation and putting it back on the rails when it starts to deviate or degenerate down a less healthy path. But hopefully you can slowly fade more into the background as the meetings progress and the group starts to find itself, growing its own identity organically. If the leader had all the answers and could solve all the problems, they would not need the group in the first place. Each group will develop its own identity with time, and you have a central role in the process.

Another core element for your group is honesty. This is not to say that people are naturally dishonest, but perhaps honesty, like everything, can be seen on a spectrum: some people are more wed to the truth than others. Or sometimes they feel that they're truly being honest but actually have a different impression or memory of events. I like to be explicit about the importance of honesty – it's not always stated outright as a core value, and it could be seen as a throwaway comment (of course everyone values honesty, right?), but if you're explicit about it then everybody knows where you stand, so that if issues with honesty come up in the future, it's been discussed and agreed upon. I refer again to the base of Patrick Lencioni's pyramid in *The Five Dysfunctions of a Team*: TRUST. Without honesty, the group will not have trust in each other. Trust develops over time, but without a uniform embracing of honesty, it may not develop at all. Remember, you want your group to get into the weeds, to have conversations that involve some touchy or controversial issues, as those are where the tension points are that you have to work through on your way to achieving your overarching goals. They need to be prepared prior to hitting those tension points, and that preparation involves having trust in each other that they can have a difficult conversation and still respect one another. Actually, if done well, you can come out of the difficult conversations feeling even better about the group, knowing that they had the maturity and trust to come through it healthy and stronger.

What other qualities do you want to imbue in your group, or at least consider? Another I would suggest is embracing the diversity of the group. Although we are naturally drawn to people who are like us and share similar personality traits, most groups function better when there are divergent ideas and perspectives, and when these are not only accepted but celebrated. If you can set the tone early – that you want the group to be not only active but proactive, to expect diversity and potentially some conflict – people will be more accepting when it occurs and be more open-minded. But again, it does not come naturally or quickly for most groups, so the earlier you can emphasize the importance of diversity, the more success your group will have. Not every group will need a wide range of diversity, either of members or thought, but most will benefit from it; having your members embrace it early is key.

What Are Acceptable Behaviors, and What Are Not?

With these concepts in mind, let's think a little about which behaviors you'll accept in the group and which ones might be detrimental. We already mentioned the double-edged sword of humor – you have to carefully monitor how it's used, being mindful not just of content but also of style. For example, sarcastic humor has a strong tendency to be negative and demeaning, and usually is incongruent with team building. I tend simply to point these things out when they occur the first time so we can all learn from them, but sometimes you'll find a team member who more frequently makes potentially damaging comments or jokes, likely necessitating a bit of direct counseling.

All team members want to feel respected and valued. We've talked about respect, but feeling valued is also important and needs to come from the team, especially from you as the leader. Often people feel like they're working tirelessly, putting a great deal of effort into a project or goal, but think that they're getting no recognition. As the leader, you can help them to feel "seen" in this work, even before the goals are accomplished and especially if they're having setbacks. This is not an "A for effort" principle; you're letting them know that you recognize the work they're putting in, that it is not going unappreciated. I think this is one of the core elements to wellness in medicine. People usually don't mind working hard – most people who go into medicine are extremely hardworking – but we all need to feel valued for what we're doing, recognized by our leadership for the effort we're putting in. This takes little time or effort on the part of the leader and goes a long way for the team member. But they should also feel valued by their fellow team members, and you can help foster that environment through your words and actions.

Some unacceptable behaviors unfortunately occur sometimes on teams, and you need to understand how to handle these. In fact, this is one of the most important leadership challenges, and people inside and outside your group will watch and take note of how you handle these adverse situations. Some clearly unacceptable behaviors include disrespect, discrimination, denigration, and harassment. Let's talk now about how to handle these.

Holding People Accountable

When you encounter a situation in which it appears there has been a negative event or behavior, I would keep in mind a few key principles: (1) remember that there are always two sides to the story; (2) handle things privately; (3) make sure you get all of the facts, and be as fair and transparent as possible; (4) have an action plan coming out of the situation, so that you can rebuild your team.

Behaviors are often a matter of perspective. The receiving party may feel disrespected, but they also may (or may not) be overreacting or misreading the intentions of the offending party. Similarly, the offending party may be completely oblivious to how their words or actions may have impacted others or may have intended to be playful or joking. It is a trap for the leader to try to get to the "truth of what really happened." There is no such thing. There is intention, perspective, and, hopefully, awareness. Each person needs to feel that their perspective has been listened to and adequately taken under consideration. Without this, regardless of the outcome, you may lose some of their faith in you as a leader. Each side needs to be heard and heeded.

Although it's tempting to get the two parties in the same room and "hash it out," that is usually not the right place to start. I suggest speaking with each party separately, doing more listening than talking, trying to understand the intention of the offend*ing* party as well as the perspective of the offend*ed* party. Try to get a sense of whether there is something more to the story – is there a history between the two? Is there a pattern of behavior in one or both of the individuals that may have led to this event/behavior? Is there some secondary motivation for either of them? As important as the event itself are the emotions behind and subsequent to the event, as those are what may leave scars and prevent healing. It all needs to be uncovered and discussed.

Take your time and digest both sides, and remember that you're not judge and jury – you're just trying to work through a situation, find out what went wrong, and help find a path forward. At some point you may need to get the two parties in the room together for a discussion with you, and you may need to explain to each separately the other's perspective. Or, if they're adult enough, have them explain their perspectives to each other, with you there to mediate. Regardless, the key is having them understand one another, even if they don't agree. If you don't get the differing perspectives out on the table and help them work it out, the situation will fester and prevent the group from moving forward. Your role is not to take sides but rather to help others see all sides to the story, bring them back to a common goal, and remind them of what values they all agreed to. Make sure you all leave the room with a resolution, whenever possible. They will be going back to the larger group, and people tend to talk about their grievances. For the health of the group, you'll want to make sure that the returning individuals are approaching the group dynamic with positivity and looking forward, goal-oriented.

What if you have a truly egregious event, where someone has crossed a red line? The most common situation I've encountered in my career, unfortunately, is sexual harassment. This can be in the form of verbal comments, such as inappropriate jokes of a sexual nature, or even inappropriate touching. Once again, you need to get the perspective of the offending party, but even if the intention was benign, this is still a crossed red line and needs to be handled accordingly. At the very least, the person may need counseling to gain insight to their comments/behaviors, best carried out by a trained professional outside of your institution and kept confidential. Sometimes people need to go to a more extensive course or program, such as those commonly provided by state medical societies, for more intensive counseling and assessment of people with disruptive behavior. Finally, sometimes people need to be dismissed, which is a whole separate challenge that we'll discuss later. But when you're dealing with a disruptive team member in medicine, just like in any field, as the leader you are required to address the situation. For me, a key moment is whether the individual agrees to there being a problem when the situation is pointed out to them, at least in a specific example, and shows a willingness to address it and learn more about it. Denial that there is a problem leads down a very different path, often with the removal of the team member.

Resetting the Team after a Negative Culture Event

Most teams are bound to have at least one negative culture event, if not many. The groups that have the most success are those that learn from these events, discuss them openly and honestly, and move forward feeling healthier and stronger. Easier said than done. Depending on the nature and delicateness of the problem, you might consider having a very open conversation about what went wrong and why (if you know). I find it particularly disarming as a leader to be the one to take responsibility for what happened: I should have set the tone better, I should have recognized warning signs that this might happen, I should have been more aware or engaged. Your team is most likely not holding you responsible in most circumstances (although they will in some), but your humility in taking responsibility empowers others to feel that they can be humble and accepting of responsibility as well. Some may feel that they "dodged a bullet" – a seemingly innocuous comment that went awry and hurt someone might be the kind of comment they can imagine they might trip up and make themselves, and they're feeling guilty about that. On the other hand, some may feel relatively defenseless and can be easily injured by the comments and actions of others. When they see you take responsibility for the overall situation, as well as the health of the group, they too feel protected and respected. Your actions in these times of crisis carry a great deal of weight.

Let's take the situation of where you have to take disciplinary action with one of the group members. As much as you try to keep these things private, word tends to get out anyway. Regardless, you still have to address the group and rebuild, sometimes without that team member, either due to administrative leave or frank dismissal. How do you handle these delicate situations?

I suggest going back to your roots. What are the overall goals of the group? What are the core values that you all agreed to? Go back to your mission and vision statement, zeroing in on some of these issues. Where did you fall off track from your core principles? Most importantly, *have the discussion* – don't assume that if you simply ignore it and move on, it will just go away. More likely, it will fester. Consider starting the conversation with this question: "What can we learn from this experience?" One of my mentors taught me this principle: Never let a crisis fail to be an opportunity. When a negative event happens to a group, you can either try to sweep it under the carpet and move on quickly, or you can use it as a learning experience, an opportunity to redefine who you are as a group. You can listen to the group and find out what they would like to see you do differently/better in the future. Even if the conversation is painful, I think it most often is necessary and will help your group to move forward in a positive and productive way. Without the discussion, trust may erode, and the team may degenerate into dysfunction.

We've been talking about the concept of accountability. Trust is at the base of the pyramid, and only with trust can you later have accountability. Everyone expects the leader to hold the group accountable. However, an exceptional group will hold *itself* accountable, each member feeling enabled and empowered to account for other group members, knowing that it is an expectation and will make the group more successful. Let me be clear, this is not commonly done in most groups in medicine. I have worked on some truly dysfunctional teams in my career, and most often people avoid holding others accountable for fear of confrontation and discord. But in those rare groups where we *did* have trust and commonly shared values and goals, accountability within the group could occur, and when it did, the group went to the next level. Again, this should be calibrated to your group, its specific goals, and the expected tenure of you in the leadership position or of the group as a whole. For example, as chief resident for a year, you know that your tenure will be short, but you'll need to have great intragroup accountability during that one year given the intensity of the environment and the strong interdependence. As a department chair, my tenure is longer (I hope!), with a mix of short- and long-term goals. I need to be patient in this less pressure-packed scenario and give time to let the group mature, develop subgroups/divisions, and bring on vice chairs, division chiefs, and other leaders in the department. There is greater complexity, but also greater opportunity!

Remembering to Embrace Diversity

I feel compelled at the culmination of this chapter to reemphasize the importance of diversity in your group. All along, when talking about group dynamics, we have been talking about diversity, equity, and inclusion. Diversity is essential to the group's success by bringing in divergent ideas and perspectives. It also gives people a seat at the table, especially people who are often deprived of those opportunities, traditionally people from underrepresented groups such as women or people of color. This is especially the case for leadership positions, so it is important to be not only *mindful* but also *proactive* when considering all qualified candidates for leadership positions within your group; go beyond inclusion to sponsorship and leadership. Equity is often a poorly understood concept, with some mistaking it for equality. But equity is different, and in your group, it requires an understanding of what traditionally has made things *inequitable* for certain groups. How has the medical system disadvantaged women and people of color historically? What *systematic* processes are in place that could apply to your group that inherently disadvantage certain groups based on their race, gender, or sexual orientation/identity?

Group exercises that have people envision what it is like to come from one of these groups can be very helpful and instructive. How often do white males, the traditional leader phenotype in medicine, go through such an exercise? Probably not very often. I have had the great advantage of having the administrative director for my department be a black woman. I was particularly lucky that we had the opportunity to lead our department in the setting of the Black Lives Matter movement, tackling racism head on. I learned a great deal through this process and continue to learn. I will never know what it is like to walk in her shoes, having myself grown up with white privilege. But that does not mean that I cannot try. Having your group go through this exercise may be very educational and teach them a lot about their misperceptions and inherent biases, and you may consider bringing in an outside consultant to talk about inherent or unconscious bias in the workplace. Even if you feel like it's not a problem for your group, it probably *is*, at least to some extent.

A particular area to focus on for diversity, equity, and inclusion is in the practice of recruiting and retaining, whether it be of faculty, fellows, residents, or students. Having a fair, equitable, and transparent process is integral, and successful groups are very explicit in their approaches to hiring and promoting. It starts by taking a look at the current makeup of your group and whether it's diverse and inclusive at baseline. If not, you need to ask yourself why? Is there a restricted pool of candidates that you and others are competing over? Does your workplace have a negative reputation in regard to treatment or advancement for people from underrepresented groups? Are there systemic processes that inherently disadvantage people of color or women? A classic example is asking a woman or a person of color to sit on one committee after another, so that there can be diverse representation on the committee. That serves the needs of the committee, but not of the individual – it is one more meeting for them to attend, for which they often get little or no credit and which takes them away from their primary passions, whether they be clinical, educational, or research, thus decreasing their productivity and in essence punishing them for their service. In medicine, we historically have not done a very good job of rewarding people for these selfless acts, protecting their time or even recognizing the hardships created. This is an example of a systemic flaw that, despite good intentions, further worsens the playing field for the woman or person of color.

Given the historical inequities and frank mistreatment of these groups, proactive leadership on this front is sorely needed. Not only do there need to be more women and people of color in positions of leadership, but more resources need to be provided by departments, medical centers, and medical schools, including direct compensation, both financially and in the form of protected time, for what is often asked of them above and beyond what would normally be asked of a white male in medicine. One recent example from within our own department: recognizing that we had zero African American faculty, we were very proactive with one of the African American residents in our program, offering him a faculty position at the beginning of his third year of residency (upon completion of his planned neuromuscular fellowship). In addition, the hospital provided resources to pay off a significant portion of his student loans, which numbered in the hundreds of thousands of dollars. I know that mine is not the only institution to do this kind of thing, but it made me extremely proud to be part of a place that truly put its money where its mouth is, to help this young, promising physician to feel valued, both at that moment and for the long term. And to hire like this from within our own department was a great signal to others that we are a "family" and truly care about career development at every stage. For more information on recruiting and retaining, see Chapter 3.

Now that we've talked about team principles and building the culture, I'd like to get into some detailed issues. One that can be particularly daunting, for both new and experienced leaders, is running an effective meeting. That is the subject of our next chapter.

Running an Effective Meeting

All too often in medicine, we sit through boring meeting after boring meeting, feeling like we're wasting time. That's because we typically are. Most meetings are not run efficiently or effectively, and very few leaders put the time and energy into running a meeting well, not only wasting the time of their audience but their own too. Without question, some meetings, or at least portions of meetings, are necessarily informative and perfunctory, such as updates on the financial situation of a department or the medical center or school. But not all meetings have to be like that, nor do all portions of a given meeting. It doesn't have to be "death by PowerPoint."

In this chapter, I will give some tips for running an effective meeting, getting the most out of your group in the process, and having the group feel not only updated but engaged, respected, and perhaps even inspired. Not that being a leader is a popularity contest, but one surefire way to avoid being *un*popular is avoiding inundating people with a bunch of boring meetings!

Getting People Engaged

In Chapter 4, we established the vision for the group, so everyone should know what they're aiming for. In Chapter 5, we described some cultural traits that can help define the group and establish chemistry. So, with these as your backbone, you've got a group that's ready to get to work. As you start holding meetings, you can tell them that you actually wish to avoid being boring (it's okay!) and want them to be truly engaged. This will make some in the group nervous or wary, others excited and ready to hear more. You can emphasize that their engagement is important so that the meetings can be a means to an end, not some meaningless requirement during which people can mentally check out for an hour. But the expectations need to be clear – the meetings will be *working* meetings; there will be discussion and problem-solving, and people are expected to participate. With this, they'll need to minimize distractions, such as cell phones, pagers, laptops . . . anything that can beep or flash and take them out of the moment. (Note that I said "minimize," as I'm well aware that many in medicine need to be available by phone or pager when on service, and emergencies do come up. But in general, most of the time, distractions can be minimized.)

When I first started as department chair, I remember sitting down with a division chief for one of our first meetings, getting to know each other. His phone watch kept dinging and distracting him, and he truly could not help himself from looking with each "ding." It was quite Pavlovian. Meanwhile, I waited patiently and kept my gaze on his face, waiting for him to make eye contact again and rejoin the conversation. I proceeded to tell him the story of my first chair when I was a junior faculty, who looked at me with piercing eyes and full attention. I would not have thought for one second to look anywhere else but back at her eyes. I explained this calmly and patiently to my division chief and saw the look on his face change. It was rare that such distractions occurred with us in the future, not because I "came down on" him, but because respectful, undistracted communication is essential to every group and every interaction. We must remember in this age of ever-increasing electronics and screens that there is no substitute for direct human interactions.

A big part of the effective meeting is having a well-thought-out agenda. Let's talk about that next.

Setting the Agenda (and Prework)

Some meetings have no agendas sent out in advance. Other meetings have no agenda at all. Both are mistakes. Everyone likes to know what to expect in a meeting and even to have a say in the agenda. So, I would suggest a couple of things: (1) solicit agenda items in advance (not that you have to incorporate all of them), and (2) send out the agenda in advance, at least by a day or so. This helps set expectations and also lets people know that the meeting is still taking place (and they're expected to attend!), in case you have a record of canceling meetings. So, this is one form of preparation.

Another important meeting prep technique to consider is prework, usually in the form of short reading assignments. Remember, people in medicine are very busy, so you can't give them a ton of homework, as they won't do it. But if you plan on having an important discussion and getting people's viewpoints, you have a choice between having them read about the topic in advance versus torturing them with a PowerPoint presentation for 30 minutes, and then having the discussion. Which do you think is more effective? Perhaps it's a revision to a clinical policy that you have them review in advance. Or perhaps it's a research proposal or the CV of a person you're considering hiring. People will get the point that you expect them to come to the meeting prepared for discussion; you don't want to be that person who is hastily leafing through the CV during the meeting, or hunting for the CV on your cell phone, while others are having a fruitful discussion.

Taking this to the next level, your agenda can take on more structure, with multiple categories of topics:

- *Inform.* These are brief presentations, not necessarily with slides, that are meant to be information only. These should be minimized to the bare essentials. (This is for required, often perfunctory information.)
- *Discuss.* These are the topics where you want to encourage a discussion from the group. Sometimes they will need to have done their prework and come prepared for the discussion based on that, whereas other times you may give a brief presentation to set the table for the discussion. For example, what is the issue the group is facing, and what are the important aspects to consider in the discussion?
- *Vote.* This can also be based on the prework or on the discussion, but this helps people to be prepared to put their money down and vote on an issue.

Once you've got these categories, another useful management tool is to put estimated times next to each agenda item: we'll spend five minutes presenting on this issue, with ten minutes of discussion and five minutes to vote. Then it's on to the next item. This helps everyone to stay focused and understand what's expected of them. Again, both children and adults need structure, and if you provide structure to your meetings, people will be happier. Oh, and by the way, start and end your meetings on time!

Another interesting and fun form of a meeting is one centered entirely around discussion, such as a brainstorming or thematic session. For example, our department's "strategy committee" held a session to discuss mentorship for the department, and I posed them six questions to consider in advance:

(1) What are the different types of mentorship (research, education, clinical, career, life)?
(2) What constitutes "good" mentorship?
(3) How do we measure the success and/or efforts of mentors? (The answer needs to involve the mentee[s].)
(4) How do we mentor the mentors to become more effective?
(5) What are the obstacles our mentors face, and how can we help them overcome them?
(6) How do we make sure that our mentorship aligns with the goals of the department and the institution as a whole?

The discussion was animated, energetic, fruitful, and inspiring. We discovered at the end of one hour that we had barely scratched the surface in our understanding of mentorship in our department, but we all realized its extreme importance, and that a thoughtful, deliberate approach would be necessary to comprehend and address mentorship responsibly in the future. It was a great discussion!

Let's shift now to some of the more challenging aspects of meetings – having a constructive discussion without it degenerating into a free-for-all, hurt feelings, or a dysfunctional group.

Establishing Trust

As mentioned in previous chapters, the trust you develop with your group will be one of its most important qualities and will dictate whether you're able to truly grow and develop together. Nowhere is this trust on greater display than in your meetings, where you're thrown into a dialogue with each other, asked to participate in an honest and earnest fashion, and may encounter some uncomfortable situations or conversations. You've got to have trust in each other to navigate through these in a healthy manner. Keep in mind that your group can probably sail along just fine in the conventional sense, by having traditional meetings with little interaction or conversation. And if that's what you're aiming for, you can probably skip ahead in this book. But what I'm encouraging is not to settle for the ordinary for your group but rather to be *extraordinary* and achieve more than you previously thought you could, by opening up to each other, learning, and growing together.

So, as with most concepts put forward in this book, I would recommend being very outward and open with your intentions. You're not going to avoid challenging concepts, you'll actually foster them and foment conversations that will bring out naturally divergent ideas, encouraging innovation of thought and approaches. All of this may lead to tension points in the conversation – and that is where the trust comes in. They have to trust you as a leader, that you know what you're doing as you lead them down this path; they also have to trust each other, that if they say something in opposition to each other that it is okay – there is still respect, and those moments are encouraged. As your group learns to trust each other more over time, not only are they able to have healthier, more constructive conversations in the moment, they *look for* opportunities to work with each other as they develop this bond. Developing their trust in the group is a great long-term investment.

Your role in this is crucial. The leader needs to be able to moderate the conversation, watching for the rough patches and helping to guide people through them. You also need to know when to let the discussion proceed, even when it's difficult, and when to cut it off or redirect. The danger is that group members can develop antipathy toward each other, the process, or you, and that's when you'll lose them. Again, redirect, reorient to the goals/mission, and help them understand that the *process* is what is going to help them achieve their mutual goals in a more thoughtful, group-oriented way.

Fostering Constructive Dialogue

How do you foster the constructive dialogue you crave? First, your agenda has set the stage – people know your expectations and what is going to be discussed. Second, your prereading will get them some sense of the issues and the controversies around them. Third, be intentional. It is okay to say, "Now is where I'd like us to get 'into it' a little, tackling this difficult subject." Let's use an example: you have enough money for one strategic hire for your department at the current time, and you're torn between hiring an outstanding stroke doctor, who is a renowned clinician and educator, versus a highly talented lab researcher, who is working on mouse models for Alzheimer's disease. For the sake of argument, let's say they will cost, in total, roughly the same to bring to your department. Also for the sake of argument, let's say that you truly haven't made up your mind on which direction to go with this and want the group's input.

You have put a somewhat controversial subject on the table: choosing between a clinician and a scientist, an educator versus a researcher. Automatically, people may start putting value judgments on the individuals, feeling that one might be "better" than the other. You can help guide the conversation toward fleshing out why one might be more appropriate than the other, at this time and in the future, for your department. What are the pros and cons of each candidate or phenotype? What are the pros and cons of bringing them in now or not? Will the stroke service be in dire straits without this new doc? Will the department miss a great opportunity by not hiring this basic scientist doing important work in the field of neurology? It might be good to create lists of pros and cons for each, letting group members shout out for each category for the two candidates. Again, get them involved, have them develop the list, and then you can look at it together. The more people use their voices in these group settings, the more empowered they'll feel to be an active participant moving forward.

Let's say Nancy, one of the scientists of your group, says something slightly edgy, like "I think basic science has taken a back seat in this department long enough. Our research rankings have slipped, and we need to do something. Hiring the mouse model scientist is the right move to make at this time." How do you handle Nancy's comment? Is it inflammatory? Does it have more than a little truth to it? Does it help the conversation? I would recognize and applaud that the member has stuck her neck out a little, which may have been difficult for her, and that the point she raises is important. She is clearly trying to advocate for what she feels is a neglected group or entity, the research in the department, and is giving an important perspective. Could she have made the statement in a softer manner? Sure, but she didn't, and that may be sending another message – this issue has not received enough attention historically, and research needs better representation in this department.

The long list of suppressed grievances is coming out, and that's eventually a good thing. The researchers are now finding their voice.

Just make sure that voice does not shut down the conversation entirely. Recognize the strength of the statement, and ask the group if anyone wants to respond to it. In that challenging moment, especially as your group is just getting off the ground, no one may have the courage or desire to speak, so you may need to step in to give a contrary view, using data to respond in a respectful and affirming way to the research advocate who spoke up. Hopefully, with time, your group will appreciate the balance of the argument and feel enabled to speak up in a similar way to advocate for the clinician-educator, so that both perspectives are heard and the issue is adequately fleshed out.

So, let's now say that the issue has been examined, you've listed all of your pros and cons, and there's no more argument to be made. Can you reach consensus? Of course, the choice of who to hire and how to use limited resources may ultimately be yours as the leader, but you still want to get group buy-in and understanding for why one choice was made over another. Remember, there's a difference between consensus and agreement. Agreement implies that the group agreed to a certain path, whereas consensus is slightly different; with consensus, not everyone has to agree, but all feel that their voices and points of view were heard and respected, and they understand the ultimate decision, even if they don't agree with it. Everyone can move on to the next task, trusting more in the process, feeling that not only do they have a voice, but that it will be heard and valued.

The "No Asshole" Rule

Sticking with the case example above, let's say one of the clinicians in the group, Jim, a member of the stroke service, speaks up and says in response to the researcher, "That's just like you, Nancy, only thinking of yourself and the precious research community. You guys really have it easy; when do you ever take call or have to come in in the middle of the night to treat a sick patient? You get to sit in your comfy office, writing grants and papers, and by the way, get nice promotions much faster than the average clinician. That's so rich of you to advocate for yet another deadweight researcher for this department." This violates what I like to call the "no asshole" rule. What makes this statement different from Nancy's above? After all, Jim is also advocating for his group and giving his own perspective, which you've tried to encourage. He's even become passionate in the process, which is not necessarily a bad thing (it does show engagement!). There are several problems: (1) the attack became personal, (2) there was sarcasm in the comment, which will not work in this situation, (3) so much negativity – Jim was not advocating *for* a person or type of hire; he was advocating *against* a hire and, furthermore, attacking a group represented by the potential research hire. Now, his intentions may have been noble, and he may have been speaking out of pent-up frustration as well. But how do you think Nancy feels after those comments? What is going through the minds of the rest of the folks in the room? You can bet the tension is pretty thick!

There is a time for the leader to step back and see how the group handles the situation, but this is probably not one of those times. A comment of this nature does require a response, and likely from you as the tone-setter and person responsible for running a constructive conversation and meeting. I would start with some degree of validation and recognition of the value of the comment: "Jim, I appreciate your passion on this issue and recognize how you're trying to advocate for your group, which is noble and important." Everyone knows there's a "but" coming, and although Jim has been put on warning by this first sentence, he feels somewhat validated. You continue: "And as much as I want to foster a good healthy discussion around controversial issues, I need to remind the group that we have some core principles that need to be heeded. Specifically for this instance, I would emphasize the importance of avoiding personal attacks, eliminating sarcasm, and keeping to comments of a constructive, goal-oriented nature." Your tone with Jim is not only calm and patient, but it's also firm and clear. The "no asshole" rule has been violated, either intentionally or unintentionally, and the group needs to hear you call it out. Without your intervention by way of a public display of leadership and defense of a constructive conversation and diversity of opinion, the group will shut down and find escape in their cell phones, and you will have an uphill battle recovering from that meeting.

What do you do with Jim after the meeting? A separate and private conversation is warranted. Jim is not necessarily an asshole himself, but his comments violated the rule. What were his motivations? What was he thinking in the moment? Does he have insight and regret for the comments? I would suggest opening that conversation with, "Tell me your thoughts about that meeting." What Jim does in this moment will be crucial for his future in the group, and he could take it in a variety of directions. But you asking him for his perspective at the outset tells him that he has an opportunity to share his experience and that (hopefully) his viewpoint will be respected. Depending on his motivations and insight, Jim may be able to return to the table and have a healthy relationship with the group. Sometimes an apology may be necessary, for Nancy in particular, for the group as a whole, or for both. But sometimes Jim really is an "asshole," and you'll have to decide whether and how to rehabilitate him. We'll discuss this in Chapter 8.

Wrapping It Up, Next Steps

The end of the meeting is almost as important as the beginning but is most often neglected, particularly if no time is saved for a wrap-up, discussion of things accomplished in the meeting, and next steps. Try to save a few minutes at the end of each meeting with your group for a brief recap (if it's very brief, no one will mind if a meeting ends early!). Go back through the items on your agenda, noting the results of votes and discussions and where loose ends still exist. If there is "homework" or action items from the meeting, or subgroups that have been formed to tackle a particular issue, reiterate what the tasks are and the expected timeline for completion and reporting back to the larger group. Give your group a sense of where they're making progress toward their goals and where this meeting fits in with the grand scheme of things. Give the meeting *pertinence* from beginning to end. The group will feel a sense of accomplishment and purpose and will be more likely to come to the next meeting ready to be engaged.

Finally, send out minutes. This can be in the form of crude notes from the meeting taken by you or someone else designated to do so and should follow the agenda items. Not everyone will necessarily read the minutes, but, again, it's good to have these points of reference in case they're needed in the future. The group will see you as organized, goal-oriented, and invested in their success. Their faith in you as a leader is growing, as is their faith in each other.

Special Meetings: A Retreat

If your team is running into a funk, or perhaps you need a reset to refocus your agenda or goals, a retreat can be a very valuable tool to bring the team back together and energize it. There are many models for retreats from several industries that can help, and there is no "one size fits all." But there are some general principles that may be helpful to you as you go through this all-important exercise.

First, consider the venue, timing, time, and facilitator. I'm a strong proponent of off-site retreats, as there are too many distractions in our daily workplace, and you want people to be fully engaged during the retreat. You want it to be a place that is relatively easy to travel to, as we all have busy lives. It can be somewhere scenic (e.g. an ocean view) or famous/inspirational (e.g. Gettysburg), but remember, you're not there for the scenery but rather to reengage with each other. Often, a hotel boardroom will work just fine, and it takes care of meals, coffee, and so on; they often have a clear understanding of what's needed in addition, such as an appropriately sized room for the group you bring, a table and chair set-up for facing each other for discussion, wall space for sticky notes, and so on. As for the timing, given that in medicine we tend to have very busy days early in the week, a Friday may be best, even knowing it will impact the finances a little. Weekend retreats are tricky, as they take people away from their families, and they will feel guilty saying no; best to avoid. The time devoted can be a half-day, full day, or two days, depending on your needs and what you'd like to accomplish. The facilitator is key – it can be you, as the group leader, and this can certainly cut down on expense. But it's usually best to use someone from outside the group who has experience running successful retreats, as most of us in medicine do not, and people don't like wasting their time. Remember, many people come into retreats already rolling their eyes and looking at their watches; you want to utilize the time smartly, engaging and invigorating them, rather than having them resent you for putting them through the process.

The next step is the prework: what do you want your group to read or think about prior to the retreat? It's useful to give them an agenda ahead of time so they know what to expect, as well as to have input into it. You may also wish to provide one or two short pieces to read that are pertinent to the exercise, perhaps around team building, goal setting, or conflict resolution, whatever will be the main subject of the retreat. You might even have some key members of the group meet with the facilitator ahead of the retreat, in order to set expectations, enlist their help, or prep them for topics that may be challenging for them. With a little bit of prework, you can turn curmudgeons and naysayers into active participants and perhaps even champions for the retreat.

At the retreat itself, there are several key principles that you may find effective. First, it can be a great opportunity to get reacquainted on a personal level. I don't mean getting into deep, dark personal secrets, but rather what are people's motivations? What do they find rewarding about their work? Why did they choose this path? What do they hope to get out of working with this group? This need take no more than three to five minutes per person and is a really valuable way for people to see the best in each other again and understand where they're coming from. It sets the table for the bigger items on your agenda, which should be goal-oriented. Pick one or two (more becomes unwieldy) specific problems you'd like the group to tackle, both important for the group but also tangible and digestible. There can be some controversy around the topics (e.g. reorganizing the goals of the group), or they can be more strategic (e.g. setting three- and five-year milestones). But they should be inherently of obvious importance to the whole group, so that they understand why they need to work on it. You can break into smaller working groups that report back to the larger group – this helps not only with workflow but also team building. At the culmination of the retreat, recap what you've accomplished and be very specific. Help the group to see how the retreat was part of the overall process and will inform their more routine, day-to-day work and meetings.

Don't forget to have follow-up to the retreat. Survey the group to find out what they liked or would do differently next time. Ask them how the retreat should inform the interactions of their group in the future and whether/when to do the next retreat. And don't forget to give your impressions of the retreat as the leader of the group, what you took from it and what you'd like to see from the group moving forward. They will be interested in your thoughts in particular, and how you've incorporated the new knowledge gained into the group's future. It's a great way to bring it home.

Now that you've oriented your group, set goals, and started to develop your personality, both as a group and as a leader, let's shift gears. The next chapter will be about aligning goals with administration in medicine, both the hospital and, for those in academic medicine, the medical school.

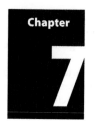

Aligning Goals with Hospital and Medical School Leadership

Whether you lead a small group, a division, a residency, or a department, aligning with the goals of the hospital and medical school are essential to ensuring your group's success. All too often, we see the leadership above us as obstructionist, miserly, or otherwise misguided or misaligned. This is usually not the case, in fact, but there are often communication issues up and down that create that impression and sometimes lead to an adversarial relationship. Both groups benefit by aligning their goals, and the earlier they do so, the better.

This chapter will speak mostly to aligning your goals with that of your hospital, with some time at the end devoted to the medical school. They have many similarities but some important differences. Understanding their priorities will help you to align yours.

Financial: Understanding Their Resources and Yours

I have worked at multiple hospitals during my career, including University of Florida, Massachusetts General Hospital, Brigham and Women's Hospital, Yale New Haven Hospital, and now Boston Medical Center. Regardless of the place or time, hospital administration would unfailingly say each year that "we're facing a particularly challenging year financially, and we're all going to have to do our part to get through it." Although it is a bit humorous to hear this every year, I don't believe that it is actually dishonest; hospital administrators do face enormous challenges every year, and even if the year ends up better than expected, the healthcare landscape changes so much each year, at least in the US, that it is hard to keep up and pivot to new rules and regulations that often seem almost designed to make healthcare less profitable. And the doomsday scenario is always lurking – the multimillion dollar lawsuit, major changes in billing and compensation guidelines for a previously profitable program, or, as happened without warning in 2020, the global pandemic. For hospitals that are truly just skimming by, these can be catastrophic events, one for which they may have no answer.

From a leadership perspective, you will benefit from taking this into account when working with your hospital on funding programs, understanding that they are in fact not a money tree and that you need to be seen as part of the solution rather than some whiny, obtuse, self-serving thorn in their side. Most hospitals will present their financials frequently, sometimes monthly; this is certainly the case for most chair groups. Often the presentations include comparative data specific to each department, so you can see how your department is performing relative to others on a given metric. My advice to you is to pay attention to what they're presenting – the more educated you are about their finances and your performance, the less tone-deaf you'll appear when you're looking to collaborate with them on program development, a strategic hire, or an important project. Sure, spreadsheets are boring, but they're also informative, and if you have a good administrative director, it behooves you to pore over this data with them to understand the overall finances as best you can.

Likewise, have a sense of what your own finances are and what your sources of funding can be. If you're a department chair, you usually start out with some type of "chair package," which can vary in size greatly depending on the department and the institution. But whether your package is big or small, try to gain a deeper understanding of what it is intended to be used for and what gets funded through other mechanisms. For example, you may get a very large package but are expected to pay rent for your clinic use every year from this fund, which is essentially paying a hospital expense and forcing you to design and utilize your clinic space wisely (not necessarily a bad incentive); this could be considered a hyperinflated package. On the other hand, you might have a more meager package, but many expenses are already covered by the hospital (or medical school), thus lessening your overall needs. For example, for new hires, the hospital might backstop their clinical shortfall for some period of time while they're ramping up their practice, and you'll only be expected to cover their academic time (e.g. research or education). Rather than looking at the total dollar amounts, you have to understand how things work at your institution – they're all different, so take the guesswork out of it and just ask. Usually you'll have a hospital VP who is designated to work through these issues with you, and they'll likely be impressed that you, as a physician leader, want to have a deeper, better understanding of the finances in your domain. And they'll be looking to you for guidance as they're putting together your package – what do you foresee as the department's needs, both short and long term, what will it cost, and will it lead to a better state of financial stability and growth, for both your department and the institution?

Most places will have at least two and sometimes three sources of funding: hospital, medical school, and medical group (or physician's organization). The dynamics are always different, so I would recommend taking the time to learn the ins and outs of each, and who is responsible for what, so that you can align goals all around.

What Is Their ROI?

The hospital is constantly thinking about the ROI, or return on investment. They are continually being asked for resources for this and that, and in order for them to have an appetite to fund *your* request, they need to see the potential ROI. Your job is to come prepared, which means doing your financial homework. Although you may have the talent and gift to make a very passionate and convincing appeal, if you haven't done your financial homework you'll likely be sent back to reappear later with a sound business plan. For example, I may think that a neurorehabilitation specialist would be a great thing for our department and our patients; I might even say that it presents unique research opportunities and would complement all of our divisions in neurology, from stroke to MS to movement disorders. And all of this might be true, but if I'm unable to make a cogent and compelling financial argument, the proposal is dead on arrival.

This is not to say that every proposal has to be a moneymaker for the hospital, and of course not all will be. Sometimes you can get by with a break-even proposal, wherein at least the hospital will come out neutral. But other times you'll need to advocate for a program that will be a clear money-loser, at least for your department, and you need the hospital's support to make it work. These proposals need, at the very least, to have great strategic importance in order to get traction (e.g. increasing hospital visibility overall by advertising a new program), and they often fail on the first attempt to get support. But if the program is important to you, and you feel that it truly does align with the hospital's overall mission and goals, you can learn from the experience and come back to the table at a later time. You may also be able to convince them of other sources of revenue created by the program, otherwise known as "downstream effect," which I'll discuss next.

What Is Your Downstream Effect?

Depending on the program you're trying to build or the person you're thinking of hiring, you can consider the potential downstream effects generated for you, the hospital, the medical school, or all of the above. Consider the following scenarios:

(1) You want to hire an endocrinologist. Let's say that endocrinologist will be hired at a salary of $150,000 per year, plus fringe, costing about $225,000 in total per year. An endocrinologist performs mostly evaluation and management (E&M), and although they're full-time clinical, working eight or nine half-day sessions per week, they only generate a little over 3,000 Work Relative Value Units (wRVUs) per year – not enough to cover their salary plus fringe. But they generate downstream revenue: (a) imaging of the thyroid, pancreas, and so on; (b) pharmacy, including revenue

from infusions to treat autoimmune endocrine disorders; and (c) surgery, such as thyroid, pancreatic, and adrenal surgeries, and even highly lucrative neurosurgeries, such as transsphenoidal pituitary surgery.

(2) You want to hire a vascular neurosurgeon, at a salary of $750,000 per year, plus fringe. Given that there is adequate volume, the vascular neurosurgeon can earn their salary through their procedural volume, generating both professional and technical revenue. They also may generate downstream revenue by all of the neuroimaging they order, as well as supporting the volume of the neurocritical care unit. And one more downstream effect is helping the hospital to maintain its status as a Comprehensive Stroke Center, important for staying competitive and maintaining volume, as well as for advertising. Some of these downstream effects are calculable, while others are not as easy.

(3) You want to build a new program in dementia. A behavioral neurologist commands a salary of about $200,000 per year, and a neuropsychologist about $140,000 per year, both plus fringe. Given the nature of the beast (dementia patients require slow, patient, methodical evaluations), the behavioral neurologist can only see two to four patients in a half-day session, and the neuropsychologist even fewer – one or two – given the extensive testing they perform. They clearly will not generate their salaries with this kind of productivity, but they do generate imaging, including MRIs and even advanced positron emission tomography (PET) scans. Sometimes they generate revenue through neurosurgeries, such as ventriculo-peritoneal shunts, although this is not highly remunerative. But having an Alzheimer's Disease Center is important to the hospital – it gets them "points" on their evaluation for national rankings, such as in the US News and World Report. And Alzheimer's disease and dementia are gigantic and growing public health problems, with many ongoing clinical trials, which can also bring in revenue both to the department and to the hospital or medical school (through indirect costs). So you can make the case.

I would suggest, whether you're going to ask for financial help from hospital leadership or not, that you go through this exercise with every potential hire or program you're entertaining, as it will give you a means to track your finances and contribution margins for people and programs over the long term, always a good thing.

Understanding the Key Individuals

Regardless of where you work, there are likely multiple layers of leadership above you, on both the hospital and medical school sides, and having a keen understanding of who is responsible for what, and who to go to and when, will not only set you off on the right foot, but will also make you more efficient when you need resources and will promote good relationships up and down the food chain. You can't go straight to the CEO or dean with every concern or complaint. They expect you to work through their system, and although it's easy to complain about bureaucratic red tape, leadership structures are in place for a reason, as there has to be a division of labor and responsibility. The sooner you realize they're not "out to get me" or "trying to make life hard for me," the more effective you'll be as a leader advocating for your group.

Understanding that all medical centers are a little different, there are a few principles of organizational structure that are more common than not. As you start in your new leadership position, you might ask to see the organization chart ("org chart"), if one exists (and one usually does). If it doesn't exist, then you need to do a bit of homework and start meeting with people to gain a clearer understanding of their roles and responsibilities. Below the CEO/President of the hospital, there is typically a C-suite. This is not unique to medicine, but medical centers do have some twists to their "Cs." In addition to the CEO, there is often a Chief Financial Officer (CFO), a Chief Operating Officer (COO), a Chief Information Officer (CIO), and, in medicine, a Chief Medical Officer (CMO) (and sometimes a Chief Surgical Officer [CSO] as well) and Chief Nursing Officer (CNO). Next, there are a number of Vice Presidents (VPs), and sometimes an Executive VP who sits in the C-suite as well. VPs are often responsible for the oversight of a number of different departments and thus act as a sort of intermediary between the chairs and the C-Suite. Thus, the relationship between chair and VP becomes a crucial one. VPs also commonly work with people other than the chair within the department, including the vice chairs, business administrator (BA), and medical directors (e.g. inpatient and outpatient, depending on the department). Other key players include the Designated Institutional Official (DIO), who oversees graduate medical education (GME) for the institution, marketing/advertising directors, heads of development, a Chief Compliance Officer (also labeled "Quality and Safety"), and human resources (HR). Sometimes these positions are duplicated within the medical school, adding to your list of people with whom you are interdependent. The chair of the department becomes a great big double-sided funnel, through which information and systems flow down to the department, and clinical, educational, and research priorities flow up to the hospital (and medical school) leadership.

Clearly, chairs play an integral role in the operations and success of a medical center, but being a chair is not a solitary role. The most important relationships for the chair within their department are with the BA, vice chairs, and medical directors, closely followed by the division chiefs. But of all of these, the BA is probably the most crucial. Most physicians who become chair do not have a strong background in business administration (although more and more chairs are getting MBAs), nor do they typically have a great affinity for managing finances or even navigating spreadsheets.

It is the BA's responsibility to understand all of this and, further, to help you to gain a deep understanding of these issues. I consider the BA as coleading the department, playing a strong complementary role to the chair to make sure the finances are sound, good systems are in place, and that you're strategizing for the future. With a trusting relationship, they can even become a great sounding board (and sometimes akin to a psychologist!), although this is beyond the standard expectations, and you don't always get lucky enough to have someone with whom you share great chemistry. Business competence is essential; psychological support can be obtained elsewhere.

Establishing Trust and Common Goals

Even if the org chart is crystal clear, it might still behoove you to spend some one-on-one time with hospital leaders, especially when you first start in your role, just so you're very clear as to what they see as *their* role (not necessarily what's on paper), what they see as *your* role, and how to best communicate with that individual. Otherwise, you will be prone to misunderstandings and misconceptions, leading to frustration on both sides.

As an example, when I left Yale (where I had been serving as vice chair) and came to Boston Medical Center, my very first meeting with my VP was a disaster. I was used to one system at Yale, wherein I would negotiate for resources for projects or programs on a case-by-case basis, working with the hospital to jointly develop business plans and establish priorities for funding. I assumed that Boston Medical Center had a similar setup, and in the first meeting I asked about funding for bringing in outside speakers for grand rounds, as there was no such fund (which I found strange). This not only seemed like an innocuous request, but it was also not a large sum of money, and I thought it might be an easy, early "win" for both sides. To my astonishment, the hospital VP was highly disappointed with my request, to the point of feeling it was inappropriate. From his perspective (which was reasonable!), he had just gone through all this effort to put together a strong chair package with considerable funding, and here I was asking for even more money at our first meeting. The rest of the meeting did not get much better, and my BA (also new) and I walked out of the room forlorn and confused. We had failed to understand the perspective of our leadership, as well as how things worked at our new institution. It took many months to repair the relationship with the VP (it is repaired now, though!).

So, as you're going around meeting with the various hospital leaders to whom you'll be reporting, it's helpful to ask honest, open-ended questions, such as the following:

- "Can you please tell me a bit about your specific role, particularly as it relates to my department?"

- "How would you describe your communication style, and what works (and doesn't) when people communicate with you?"
- "For chairs and leaders who have been successful here, what has made them successful? For those who have struggled, do you have any insights as to why?"
- "What are your priorities, and how can I and my department work best with you to help achieve them?"

The answers and discussion around these questions will likely fill the hour nicely but also set the tone that you're genuinely interested in working well with them, that you're interested in aligning your goals with theirs, and that you're going to be a *good partner*. It's not like you have to become best friends and grab a beer after work; you just need to have a good working relationship.

Getting to "Plain Speak"

There's having meetings with your hospital leadership, and then there's having *effective* meetings with them. As stated above, this takes having a clear understanding of each other's roles and demonstrating mutual respect. It's easy to fall into the trap of attributing misunderstandings and miscommunications to one person being "medical" and the other "administrative/business," but that convenient oversimplification usually leads to nowhere. You've got to find common ground and a healthy way to communicate.

What I call "plain speak" is the form of communication where you no longer have to wonder about the other person's motives or agenda, getting rid of the mistrust and suspicion. It is challenging to achieve in conversations with hospital leadership, unless you've laid the groundwork described above, showing them that you're interested in what's going to be good for the institution overall and not just for your department/group. They need to see that you've thought past your own goals and that your desires to grow or reimagine a service are in alignment with the hospital's overall mission, that they are in tune with the hospital's priorities for that year (knowing that hospital budgets change on a yearly basis), and that you've thought far down the line – what will this program look like in three to five years, what will its needs be then, and what kind of ROI can the hospital expect over time? Remember, the bigger and more expensive the project, the more gun-shy hospital leadership will be, forcing you to make your case in a thoughtful, patient, and sometimes piecemeal way. They may not be able to fund the entire project this year, but perhaps they'll fund one chunk of it, then another part the following year, until over time you've built the program together in a graduated and understanding manner.

Let's say your relationship is less than perfect with your VP or CMO, despite all of your hard work and olive branches. You've done your best to show them you're trying to align goals, you've presented your business case in the soundest way possible, but they're still unwilling to budge. There are a few things to keep in mind. First, how important is what you're asking for? You have to decide if this is mission critical (really) or some degree short of that. In other words, you have to decide whether you're willing to "die on this hill." The number of hills you should attempt to die on in your career should be very, very few; if you get a reputation as a crusader who makes *every* project mission critical, you won't get much buy-in from your leadership (and you probably won't last very long in the role).

If your project or problem truly is mission critical and you're not getting anywhere with your VP/CMO, you may be tempted to go above their head to the President/CEO. This requires careful navigation, and depending on your relationship with your VP, you might just tell them that you recognize that you have a difference of opinion, that you respect their opinion, but that you'd like to appeal to the President/CEO to get their thoughts. In other words, *tell* them you'd like to go above their head and why, and that you respect them enough to discuss that move in advance. This is vital, for when you do meet with the President/CEO to plead your case, you can bet that their very next phone call or email will be to the VP to find out their perspective. As you can see, there is danger all around with this one, and appeals to the top of the food chain should be made extremely sparingly, with full disclosure and emphasis on respect for the other's position. And you have to ask yourself before all of this, are you *truly* willing to die on this hill? We often say we are, but when push comes to shove, you'd better be pretty darn sure.

Aligning Goals with the Medical School

Many of the principles discussed above for aligning with hospital leadership apply to the medical school as well, for those who work in academic medical centers. Medical schools and hospitals most often have different, sometimes competing interests, financial structures, and inputs; historically, medical schools were a strong source of revenue and support for clinical medicine, but the tables have turned in the last couple of decades, and it's now more common that the hospital is the primary source of revenue.

For your institution, you'll need to ask a few questions about how things work with the medical school:

- What is the medical school's financial status and input to clinical departments?
- How is research (clinical, translational, and basic science) divided between the medical school and hospital, and how is that determined? What are the indirect and fringe rates?

- What support does the medical school provide toward funding the educational mission?
- Does the medical school provide administrative support to clinical departments?
- Who are the key players and what are their roles?

There is also a separate org chart for the medical school; the head is typically the dean, followed by several assistant or associate deans, including those responsible for faculty affairs, education, research, and administration. It is important to remember that deans themselves also report to someone, typically the president of the university (or a board of trustees, or both), who may be ultimately responsible for how the funds flow to or from the medical school. Their respective roles vary from school to school, so it is helpful to understand how things work at your institution.

Most medical schools have a formula for how funds are directed to clinical departments, comprised of educational, research, and administrative contributions (clinical funding is typically the responsibility of the hospital or medical group). Depending on the school, a large amount of funding may come from medical student tuition or state funding to support medical education, thus helping to support the efforts of clinical educators in your department, such as your clerkship directors and administrative staff; however, this funding is almost always inadequate, and department chairs are often left to scramble to cobble together funding to protect the time and effort of clinical educators.[1] Sometimes, there is a structure in which the clinical revenue of the department supports "pure" educators, such as for neuroscience courses, which are often taught by nonclinician PhDs, some of whom may have lost their research funding and are dependent on this salary support. In order to avoid tension from the clinicians over these arrangements, it is important to be upfront about the integral role these individuals play in educating students, helping to create a pipeline of future clinicians that may go into their specialty. Otherwise, resentment can build.

Research funding is often a bit more complex, depending on the relationship with the hospital. At some institutions, the medical school will fund the research portion of the physician-scientist's salary, with the hospital funding the clinical effort, making the clinician beholden to both for salary support. Another model is that research is done either through the medical school or the hospital, with separate research infrastructures. Some departments may perform their research through the medical school and others through the hospital; there might even be a situation in which individuals within the same department perform their research through one or the other based on some arbitrary distinction, such as what "space" the person sits in (hospital versus medical school). The reason there are so many models out there is that there really is no perfect model – most hospitals and medical schools continue to do a strange dance with each other around research in particular, and the researchers are often caught in the middle. The goal of the leader is to gain as clear an understanding of the rules and quirks as possible, communicate this effectively with their group, and advocate for change when needed, often in collaboration with other medical leaders, such as a chair group.

Let's now dive into one of the most challenging parts of being a leader in medicine – having difficult conversations.

Note

1. D. M. Greer, J. Moeller, D. R. Torres, M. Soni, S. Cruz, L. Tornes, H. Patwa, L. Gutmann, R. Sacco, and S. Galetta, "Funding the educational mission in neurology," *Neurology*, 96.12 (March 23, 2021): 574–82.

Chapter

Having Difficult Conversations

One of your biggest challenges as a leader is having difficult conversations with members of your group. These conversations may be necessary for a variety of reasons: (1) they might be underperforming or out of compliance with documentation or billing; (2) they might have conduct that is detrimental to the team; or (3) they seem to be struggling with the team concept and the overall goals of the group. Or they may have a combination of all of the above and more. I would suggest that, in addition to leading your group effectively and efficiently, your success as a leader will be determined primarily by how well you conduct one-on-one meetings, working with "problematic" group members to help them be successful or to find a different path for them, sometimes even "managing them out." One of my favorite sayings is, "If you take in a wounded dog and nurse it back to health, it will be faithful to you forever." Not that your team's or any member's faithfulness to you is the goal; the point is, sometimes they're trying to tell you something: they're struggling and need help.

Thus, not all one-on-one meetings are punitive (in fact, most should *not* be), but they may be perceived as such, maybe by you but especially by the team member who has been "called into the principal's office." Some of this perception may be unavoidable, but part of your success for these meetings will come from your ability to portray yourself as a benevolent leader who wants to help the team member and the team alike – you have a job to do, and the number one priority always has to be team success and achieving mutually agreed-upon goals.

Setting Up the Meeting

Your prework for one-on-one meetings will dictate a great deal of what happens in the meeting, starting with how you communicate with the person that you want to meet with them. If you send an email (or worse, your assistant sends the email) that you "would like to meet with" them, but without any other explanation, their mind will quickly go to a dark place and assume the worst. That may be the case (that it *is* the worst), but it may also be something far short of that. Regardless, putting some context and reasoning into the meeting will help set expectations and frame the goals. Otherwise, the classic "Dr. X would like to meet with you ASAP. Please contact our office immediately to set up a time" can be quite terrifying, making it much less likely that you'll have a productive conversation with what will likely be a scared and very defensive team member.

A better approach would be the following email:

> Dear Dr. ——, I was hoping we might speak about what happened in the group meeting today. For whatever reason, the discussion seemed to veer off target, and I was actually concerned about some of the comments made, which could be counterproductive to the team and our goals. I would love to get your perspective on this and would greatly value your insights. I realize there are always two sides to the story, and I would like yours. Let's try to meet in the next couple of days.

This email makes it clear that you were not pleased with what happened in a group meeting (the context or event), but that you're open-minded and want to give them the benefit of the doubt as to their role in the event. It also makes it clear that there were multiple people in the room, that there's always a group dynamic, and that these conversations never really occur in isolation. You've shown that you respect different perspectives, including theirs, and want to get to the root of the matter. But you've also made it clear that you're holding them responsible, like everyone else, and that you're taking this seriously. So, with your "shot across the bow," you've also emphasized that the process will be fair and balanced. Whether the other person hears or understands any of this, well, that you can't control.

Also worth considering is where to meet – usually it will be in the leader's office, but sometimes you might go to the other person's office, so that they can feel less threatened, or even meet at a neutral site, such as over coffee, being mindful that if you're going to have a difficult conversation you will need to be in a private, quiet place. But the choice of setting sends a message as well, depending on the nature of the meeting.

Have a Plan – and a Plan B, C . . .

You know *why* you want to have the meeting with the individual, but have you thought about *what* you want the outcome (or potential outcomes) of the meeting to be? It is very helpful to have thought through the different potential scenarios in advance, so that you can steer the conversation as well as control your own emotions and responses. Are you carrying emotional "baggage" into the meeting? How do you feel about the group member? Are you frustrated, angry, disappointed, or confused? Remember, you can't control their emotions and responses, but you can control yours. Putting yourself in the right mindset prior to the meeting, as well as anticipating their potential responses (and what emotions they might trigger in you), will make you much better prepared for the meeting and allow you to navigate to a successful outcome in a healthier way, psychologically speaking.

Depending on your knowledge of the person and their personality, you might anticipate that they will react to the conversation in a variety of ways. The most common responses are defensiveness, denial, and projection, that the problem or miscommunication was someone else's fault (maybe even yours!). Sometimes, people express tremendous guilt, paralyzing them and preventing them from moving forward with the conversation in a constructive manner. Whatever feelings they are expressing, it may be helpful to recognize and acknowledge them, thus helping defuse the situation: "I understand you are shocked and angry about this, and that is understandable. I'd like to help with this situation, as these kinds of miscommunications or misconceptions are usually easily remediable." Sometimes, a group member can be sad and tearful, and you've got to be prepared to handle that as well. It may make you inclined to avoid further discussion on the subject, but this might lead to a failure to fully address the problem. If they try to deflect to others, stating that it is their fault, you can emphasize that you're trying to get all angles and perspectives on the problem and that you're saving "judgment" for now. Of course, all of this depends on the nature of the problem, and some more serious offenses (e.g. discrimination or harassment) may require a more direct approach.

I find it helpful to play out multiple scenarios. If they respond with anger, how will I react? If they respond with tears, deflection, or defensiveness, what will I do? What if they say little or nothing in response, but their body language is saying something else – what should I say? You need to have an understanding of your own mental state going into the meeting as well and whether you're carrying any emotional baggage into the conversation. How do you feel about this individual? Do they recurrently "get under your skin" and make you frustrated? Do you have a positive or negative impression of them overall? Do you have a history with them? Perhaps you rose up in the ranks while they were "left behind" when you achieved your position? Again, you can only control your emotional response, not theirs, and playing out multiple scenarios and taking your own emotional pulse may be helpful prep for a difficult 1:1 meeting.

Although it rarely comes up, sometimes you need to think of the "doomsday" scenario, in case something goes very badly in the meeting. I have actually had meetings with people who I considered mentally unstable and potentially dangerous with police or hospital security nearby, in case the person became violent or I felt that the discussion was escalating in an unhealthy and potentially violent way. Fortunately, these situations are rare, but if you consider that the person may react in an irrational and threatening manner, better safe than sorry.

Who Needs to Be in the Room?

Along the same lines, consider the dynamics of your 1:1 meeting and whether it should be just the two of you in the room together. Remember, there is already a power dynamic, as you are their leader, in a position of relative authority. There could also be other social dynamics, such as gender, race, socioeconomic status, or something else, which could make the situation extremely uncomfortable for one or both people. Think about these things in advance, and consider the optics of, for example, a senior white male leader meeting with a team member who is nonwhite and/or female, or who other-wise feels particularly threatened by the space between them and you. Don't assume that, just because your intentions are "good," there isn't a perception on the other end that you're using your power to exert control over them in some way.

Thus, it may be wise to consider having a second person in the room or at the very least leaving the office door open so that there is some semipublic aspect to the meeting, although this is often not possible given the usually sensitive nature of the subject matter. If you are resolving conflict between two team members, you can consider having both there with you at the same time, so that you and they can hear each other's points of view; however, this may also change the dynamic of the conversation, causing team members to voice their viewpoints in a different manner than if the other person was not there. You'll need to tailor your conversation, and who is in the room, to the nature of the problem and the potential complications of a private 1:1 meeting between you and them alone.

Nuts and Bolts of the Meeting

There are several principles that can help you through a challenging meeting with a team member. First, remain calm and patient. Becoming emotional or angry will never be effective in these meetings – as the leader you need to maintain control of your emotions and comportment. Second, be aware of body language, both yours and theirs. Defensive postures include crossing one's arms, glaring, and heavy breathing/sighing. Avoid eye rolling, and be careful even with smiles or other gestures that can send mixed messages. Third, spend more time listening than talking. It can be tempting as the leader to try to force the conversation in a particular direction, especially early on. Start with open-ended questions, such as "Can you tell me your impressions about that conversation?" or "Can you tell me what you meant or were thinking when you said ——?" Allow them to tell their side of the story without interruption (except for clarifications). Fourth, maintain control of the conversation by asking more directed questions as the conversation progresses, such as "Could you see how your statement could be misinter-preted?" or "Do you understand why —— might have been hurt by that comment?" Try to get the individual to gain additional perspective, including yours. Finally, in the end, be explicit in your summation of the "findings" from the meeting. For example, you might say, "I think it will be important for you to keep in mind how your words and actions can impact others" or "I hope you understand that, although your intention may have been good or benign, this behavior was detrimental to the team for these reasons, and I will be monitoring future meetings closely to make sure this is not an ongoing problem."

Consider whether the meeting should come to a final resolution. Or is it a step in the process to get multiple sides of a story, so that there will need to be follow-up meetings? And be explicit with this – by doing so, you're setting expectations and timelines; you're letting the team member know that you're going through a process – here's where you are on the timeline, and here's what the next steps will be. If, however, the meeting contains the resolution, you'll need to be very clear and calm in your presentation of your summation, why you have come to a specific conclusion, and what this means for the team member going forward. Sometimes, it's simply monitoring of the behavior moving forward; other times, it's some form of remediation or counseling; sometimes, dismissal is warranted. If you're considering the latter two scenarios, it might be good to have your supervisors aware that you're having this discussion, as well as HR and perhaps the legal team, depending on the nature of the discussion.

In my experience, most hospital and medical school HR and legal staff are very well versed in the common issues that face physicians, which include behavioral issues, alcohol or drug intoxication, or cognitive impairment. Some state medical societies have programs for evaluating impaired physicians, including the use of psychology, psychiatry, and neuropsychology. This is most commonly done in a very private process, but you and the referred clinician should be aware that the process may become part of their employment record, which may be a strong deterrent to their cooperation in the remediation.

Documentation

Carefully document the conversation, including a detailed accounting of what was said by whom. I tend to use a Word document for this and send it by email so that there is an electronic record of what was said, by whom, and when. You can ask the other party to type up the documentation or, alternatively, if there is a third person in the room, it might be part of their job to take notes. But I usually find it easiest to do this myself, giving me the opportunity to document not just what was said but what the next steps will be. Ask the other party to review the documentation very carefully and provide their edits and feedback where they disagree or had a different impression of the conversation. But make sure they know they need to respond, even if very briefly, to say they approve the meeting minutes, and save this response as part of your documentation. You are not only keeping track of what was said and when; you're creating a "paper trail" in case you need to take more formal action in the future, such as going down the path of dismissal. The more documentation you can accrue in this regard, the better.

Follow-Up

It is not enough to just document the meeting; you should always provide clear next steps and arrange follow-up. When will you touch base again, and what will be the subject of that meeting? What do you anticipate will lead to final resolution of the problem, if you know? Have the other person understand that this is a process that can go in either direction – either there is change, and they assimilate back into the group in a healthy manner, or they need to leave the group and pursue another path. There usually is no middle ground; if you allow negative or destructive behavior to continue in your group, people will lose faith in you as a leader, your group will fail to accomplish its goals, and the overall experience will be much more negative for everyone. As painful as it can be sometimes, resolving difficult team interactions is essential to the success of the group and is where you show your true mettle as a leader.

Special Consideration: Removing Someone from a Leadership Position

One particularly challenging issue is removing someone from or replacing them in a leadership position. This need to make a change can be for a number of reasons. The leader may have become ineffective or uninspired, losing their ability to rally their group. There may be someone else in the group who is chomping at the bit for the opportunity to move into the leadership position, who may leave if you don't make the change. Or the leader may be problematic, hurting the group through their actions (or inactions). The problem is compounded by the fact that most people in leadership positions carry a bit of pride or ego in having attained the position, and being forced out rather than leaving on their own terms can be very hurtful. The situation needs to be dealt with carefully and sensitively.

A guiding principle should be: take your time. Hopefully you have periodic, scheduled meetings with your leaders, whether they be division chiefs, medical directors, or vice chairs, in which you go over standard topics. Since you have these meetings with all of your leaders, the leader you're looking to replace will not feel singled out. Use these opportunities to be very clear about expectations, metrics, and timelines. Be unabashed in letting them know where and when they're coming up short, so that they're not surprised to hear they're not meeting your expectations. If there are behavioral issues, that's trickier. Come back to the culture and agreed-upon principles of good communication, and be explicit about where their behavior is deviating. Provide concrete examples from your observations or reports from others, and afford them the opportunity to respond and acknowledge the perceptions. But be clear about what conduct is beneficial versus detrimental to the team, and use the opportunity to reemphasize that your primary obligation is to the success of the greater team, and that no individual is more important than the group. Remember, you're reminding *yourself* of this as much as the leader you're looking to replace; you may hurt your relationship with this individual, but the team will be better for it in the long run, and that's where your responsibility lies.

Next, let's evaluate leadership in a crisis. You may have felt that that was the subject of this chapter, but thus far we've dealt mostly with internal pressures. Sometimes, you're thrust into a role you never expected, such as leading through a pandemic that hits the medical community harder than anything previously.

Leadership in a Crisis

In late 2019/early 2020, the coronavirus pandemic struck the globe. This was a challenge unlike any previously faced in modern healthcare and posed immense and specific challenges to leaders in the medical field. At the time of writing, the pandemic is still ongoing, but we have learned many lessons that will likely prove highly valuable for the future. This chapter will elucidate some particularly informative processes and results. While a pandemic is not the only type of crisis one might face in medicine, it is particularly illustrative, and many of the principles will apply to other types of crises. In fact, during 2020–2021, there were multiple concomitant crises that compounded the already dire situation, including the Black Lives Matter (BLM) movement and the insurrection at the US Capitol on January 6, 2021. The pandemic alone was sufficient to produce tremendous strife and agony for those working in medicine; compounded with racial inequities and injustice, as well as a horrendous insult to a precious and sacred symbol of democracy, well, it was a very difficult time.

Difficult times are when leaders need to rise up. There is no more important or impactful time for you to demonstrate your character and mettle, no time your group needs you more. Leaders cannot shrink from this responsibility, or they should be replaced. Thankfully, it does not take tremendous intelligence to strive in a crisis, but it does require character, fortitude, and courage. In this chapter, I will outline some principles that may be of use in the event of a crisis.

Understanding the Scope of the Problem

An important first step in any crisis is gaining an understanding of the scope and degree of the problem. Some crises leave you little time for this, such as the Boston Marathon bombing in 2013, in which an emergency medical situation occurred suddenly and without warning. The coronavirus pandemic gave more lead time than this, spreading over weeks from China to parts of Europe and the US, an insidious progression that seemed almost unreal and unbelievable, as well as inevitable. Over time it became quite apparent that this was going to be a global viral infectious disease event of historic proportions, similar to that of the 1918 Spanish Flu pandemic. Warning signs had been present for years, with relatively smaller viral outbreaks such as Ebola, H1N1 Influenza A, and Severe Acute Respiratory Syndrome (SARS), but these had not grown to epidemic levels, much less pandemic.

A danger for the leader is to "cry wolf" and make more of a crisis than it ends up being. However, I would argue that the danger may be far greater in making the opposite mistake, failing to see the crisis on the horizon, thus leaving your group unprepared for what is to come. Thus, a leader will best serve their group by gaining as thorough an understanding of the scope of the problem as possible, including the specific ways in which they may be affected. For a clinical department in the coronavirus pandemic, this entailed several principles: (1) keep everyone safe and healthy; (2) maintain continuity of care for the patients; (3) triage what may be deemed essential services (e.g. intensive and inpatient care) over those less essential (outpatient services), at least for some period of time; and (4) maintain the health, both physical and mental, of the group and their loved ones at home. In the early days of the pandemic, we were warned "It might last as long as two months!" Many months later, we are still fighting the disease, as well as the strain on the medical system and its workers. The mental and physical stamina this has required is indescribable.

As a leader, you can gather as much information as possible, from as many sources as you can. Information and data are empowering, and you should be as informed and up-to-date as anyone else in your group so that you can make decisions that will be timely and in their best interest.

Staying ahead of the Curve

There is a temptation to wait to be told what to do by the hospital administration and/or medical school, but as a leader, you can have a say in this as well. This is not to say that you should go rogue and counter what the hospital is saying, but remember, the larger the institution, the greater the bureaucracy and the clunkier its movements, leading to slow and often inadequate messaging. Based on your understanding of the scope of the problem, you may play a role in communicating with the administrators above you, providing gentle pushes when you feel that things may be moving too slowly in a time of crisis. How you do this is very important, as you don't want to lose your reputation or effectiveness as a good team player, but if you've got a good relationship already, you can show that you're ready to step up and be a leader among leaders.

In the specific instance of the coronavirus pandemic, it was quite clear early on that it was highly transmissible, that there were likely many asymptomatic carriers, and, by the time we were talking about it in earnest, it was probably already quite widespread in the community. We did not understand basic principles, such as when and where to wear protective masks or other personal protective equipment (PPE), or what patients might be at greatest risk. The hospital stood to lose a great deal of money by shutting down all outpatient operations, but that was clearly what was needed at that early time in order to try to gain some control of the problem and to keep our staff, docs, and patients safe. Our chair group at our hospital became quite vocal in its support of halting outpatient visits, knowing this would hurt our departments financially as well. I suspect that, due to our semipolite insistence, we were able to shut the outpatient arena down several days earlier than otherwise, perhaps sparing many infections and shifting the mindset of everyone around the hospital toward self-care, protection, and health. It wasn't just the technical aspect of stopping clinic that helped – people's thinking changed, and the seriousness of the situation was fully appreciated.

This required a rapid shift to "telehealth" visits, both by phone and video, which was a tremendous challenge worldwide. But had this pandemic happened perhaps 10 to 20 years earlier, the technology might not have been in place to even perform this ungraceful transition, so in that sense we were fortunate. Had we been more insightful, we might have seen the tremendous benefits of telemedicine long before the pandemic, but sometimes it takes a crisis to force an issue. For once, the medical system, and to some extent the US government, was able to pivot relatively quickly to continue providing care safely for millions in need. But this further increased healthcare disparities, as non-English-speaking patients or those without video capabilities (or even a phone!) were further disadvantaged, their inequities in this case broadened rather than reduced.

Communication

Communication is key in moments of crisis. Rumors start swirling almost immediately, and vast amounts of misinformation are quickly disseminated, leading to confusion, fear, and sometimes even panic. You may not have all of the information, and some of your information may not be entirely accurate. But as the leader of your group, you serve as an important source of communication in two very tangible ways: (1) your interpretation of the global information is important to your group, and (2) you can explain what pertinence the data has for your group's function. In other words, what does all of this mean for them and for the group's purpose during this time?

I have found that telling people what you know, when you know it, is extremely helpful. You may not have all of the information, and what information you have may be of uncertain veracity; that's okay, just acknowledge that, rather than propagating misinformation. It is perfectly fine to say that this information is "subject to change" or "awaiting verification," so that people can calibrate their expectations and you can maintain your reputation as a reliable source of information. Hospitals were maddeningly slow to give concrete data and information during the early days of the coronavirus pandemic, and as department chair I found that I was one of the few information sources my department trusted. But you have to make sure that you are disseminating correct information whenever possible, and that the hospital knows what you're putting out to your group.

Communication can take place in multiple settings, including in-person, via email, or through videoconferencing, for example, for faculty or division meetings. Each of these have potential pitfalls. As expected, in-person meetings are typically most effective, as you're best able to read body language and intonation of speech, but from an infectious disease standpoint, in-person is not the best idea in a pandemic, and facial expressions are particularly difficult to read when masks are being worn. Videoconferencing has become ubiquitous during the pandemic, a technology that has existed for years but had been mostly underutilized for the reasons stated above. But the benefits during the pandemic are several, including the ability to see others' faces, verbal communication, and even concomitant written communication (the "chat box"), although the latter can be quite distracting and subject to abuse. But faculty meetings, for example, are easily held over teleconference, and allow some personal touches as well. With the BLM movement, we held several department-wide town halls via videoconferencing, allowing hundreds in our department from a variety of settings to participate and share their experiences. Perhaps without videoconferencing during that time we might have remained siloed and had a very different, less meaningful conversation.

Although one might think that email communications are the least effective medium, we found them to be extremely effective during the pandemic. There are several advantages that may not be readily apparent: (1) you can take your time to put together a thoughtful and comprehensive product; (2) the recipient can choose to read the email (or not) on their own time and/or read the parts that are most pertinent to them; (3) you can provide various forms of information (e.g. updates on inpatient/outpatient operations, department finances, infection numbers, residency, and so on), organizing them into digestible factions; and (4) you can write (or quote) something inspirational! Depending on how "hokey" you are, it's an opportunity to inspire your troops and help them through a hard time. True, some of your troops may not be "hokey" themselves, but they can choose not to read that part (label it for them so they know it's coming!) or take it with a grain of salt if that's not their thing. In the end, although the emails can be a bit long, there can be a little something for everyone – data, updates, shout-outs, pictures, and inspiration.

Not all communication is good or successful, and one of my early lessons was in communicating the storm clouds on the horizon to the residents. I remember meeting with them in person the week before the pandemic hit our hospital – it was an emergency meeting, and it was quite somber. Prior to me, no one had spoken with them about what this pandemic might mean for them, the true frontline workers for highly infectious patients. Residents are already young, impressionable, and vulnerable at baseline, and I inadvertently heaped on additional stress to their lives in my impromptu speech that was designed to warn but also inspire them. I stated that this would be one of the most severe challenges of our lifetime, the likes of which we haven't seen since World War II. Although of course this ended up being true, they did not know it at the time, and they were paradoxically scared and intimidated when I had only aimed to prepare them and let them know we would be there for them. In times of stress, people will sometimes only hear the negative message, no matter your intention. After being educated after my speech by my dear residency program director, I sent a note of apology to the residents for contributing to their stress rather than alleviating it. And I let them know I was proud of them, which they needed to hear. I also think that their hearing an apology from their chair for my mistake was helpful to them, allowing them to see me as fallible and human (which I am in spades!).

Lastly, give some thought to your frequency of communications – too infrequent and people feel in the dark; too frequent and you lose your impact. In the height of the pandemic, we held faculty meetings every other week (very well attended) and division chief meetings on alternating weeks. The residency meet every week. The hospital met with the chairs every week. Early on, we sent out a weekly "end-of-the-week" email, which many commented was their favorite (and sometimes "only trusted") source of information; we later spread this out to biweekly and then monthly. Although these emails were our most effective means of communicating with the whole department, they were time- and labor-intensive, and a leader's time management during a crisis is more important than ever.

Aligning Above and Below

As mentioned earlier, keeping your message, as well as your mission, consistent with the hospital's is essential, even when they're moving slowly. They likely have more data than you, and it's better to ingratiate yourself with them by aligning with their message, rather than bucking them in a time of crisis. They are looking around for allies and team players, just like you are, and you want to be seen as part of the solution, not the problem. It's okay to agitate and advocate, but do so respectfully, always with an eye to help.

The same can be said as you look inward to the group you're leading. You need them to be on board with your plan for crisis management, so swift and clear communication is key. You don't have a lot of time to get buy-in, and you can say that upfront. Some issues will be up for discussion, and others will not. That may sound a bit heavy-handed, but most people will give you some leeway when acute decisions are needed, provided that you provide justification for hard or controversial decisions, at least at some point. That point does not need to be in the moment necessarily – it can come days or weeks later – but if it disproportionately affects one part of the group versus another, such as shutting down the neuromuscular service but maintaining the stroke service, the neuromuscular folks will need to hear exactly why at some point.

On a departmental level, crisis mode for our department required frequent (weekly) communication via videoconference with the division chiefs, vice chairs, medical directors, and residency program directors. We asked each representative to briefly give an update on activities within their domain and the current challenges they were facing. This accomplished multiple things. First, we had an idea about what was going on specifically in each area and what their needs were. Second, everyone else heard it too (or at least had the opportunity to hear it), so that everyone could have the same or similar perspective. Third, it maintained and even improved the cohesiveness and camaraderie of the group, as they had a sense that they were in it together, interdependent. The hard work we'd put into our group leading up to this was paying off; we had trust and accountability and zero infighting (at least for a time).

The second part of our weekly leadership meetings was to anticipate and discuss challenges in the weeks and months ahead, such as how could we reopen our clinic safely and what services and patients would be prioritized. We discussed challenging financial matters, such as asking senior leaders to take a temporary pay cut to help the department and institution's finances. We spoke of the need to communicate effectively, clearly, and consistently with the department, including junior faculty, residents, advanced practice practitioners, and support staff, as there is danger in mixed messaging. We discussed how to support our frontline providers – including our intensivists and stroke group – the most, not only in terms of financial support but also from the perspectives of safety and mental health. We even looked into our own avenues and connections to try to secure personal protective equipment for our department, with the blessing of the hospital. This all took a great deal of planning, input, and communication, only possible with a well-functioning group.

Education

We also needed to address how to reemphasize education during the pandemic, both for residents and students. Residents needed to understand that we were still prioritizing their education, which was not going to pause for the pandemic. Medical students were most impacted. They were actually asked to pause for several months, which had major pipeline implications, so reincorporating them back into the clinical realm was not just a "nice" thing to do – it was a necessity, not just for the students, but for the sake of the medical field moving forward.

By prioritizing the restart of our resident clinic as one of the first to come back in-person (along with electromyography and electroencephalography services, both revenue-generating for the department), it sent a strong message that we remained deeply invested in their education and recognized its importance even when they were asked to sacrifice in so many other ways, such as helping to cover the medicine services due to the sheer volume of COVID patients our hospital was caring for. Again, most residents do not mind working hard (within humane limits, of course) but need to feel "seen" and valued. They recognized and appreciated our efforts to prioritize them and maintain didactics and continuity clinic throughout.

But the educational efforts likely had a broader reach than the residents and students, with a positive effect on our faculty as well. In academic medical centers, education is part of the fabric of daily life and one of the most compelling reasons why people choose academia. By continuing education, we incorporated a sense of normalcy into people's lives – despite the tragedy and crisis all around us, we maintained a commitment to one of the core pillars of academic medicine: educating and training the next generations in our field. It became another front on the battle against the virus as well, our way of showing that life would go on despite the pandemic.

Survey, Learn, Adapt

It is tempting to think that crisis management is a one-time event, that you have this existential threat that requires spur of the moment action, and then you're through it. But crises are rarely so short-lived, and the coronavirus pandemic is a useful example of how they can be multifaceted and painfully prolonged. Naturally, your response as a leader must change, as well as your communication to your constituents. You have to ask yourself: do you really understand what they want or need to hear? How in touch are you with their needs and circumstances?

Although the value of surveys in medical science is limited and their findings usually biased, they can be quite informative when you're learning to communicate effectively with your group. They allow anonymous input from every corner, helping you to prioritize and focus your communications. We surveyed for feedback about both our faculty and leadership meetings, as well as the weekly emails to the department. Through this, we gained a better understanding of what was and wasn't working. For the most part, more data is almost always better, and even recognition of limitations in the data was appreciated (what you know, and what you recognize you don't know). We also recognized that, although the "touchy feely" parts of the emails such as inspirational words or quotes, weren't everyone's thing, for some people it was very meaningful, as it showed a warmth in the leadership that they craved. Realizing it wasn't for everyone, we actually put a semihumorous "warning" that the sappy part was next, and they could feel free to skip it!

Turning from the handling of the pandemic to the Black Lives Matter movement, we took a very deliberate and open approach not only to the discussion and venting stages but very importantly to the "action" stages as well. We held two department-wide town halls (most of our faculty are white, but most of our support staff are from underrepresented racial groups, mostly black), with intervening focused task forces. The town halls were for outlining the problem, sharing experiences, and describing our proposed approach (the first town hall) as well as progress made (the second town hall). We made it clear that we felt that talk is cheap, and without actual tangible action, as well as measurable results, we were not going to make any headway in racial inequity. Our task forces, comprised of volunteers from the town halls, focused on racial equity in (1) research, (2) clinical care, (3) education, and (4) administration. We hope that this focused approach is going to lead to tangible results for our department and that in doing so, we may serve as a model for others. Like the old saying goes, "Think globally, act locally." As a leader, you can make a difference, well beyond your own four walls.

Mental Health

We also made "wellness" a major focus for residents and students, as well as the whole department. Wellness has become a major buzzword in medicine in recent years, but it means different things to different people. As a leader in medicine, it is important to be aware of the strong prevalence of mental illness in the field, most notably depression and anxiety; this also affects some specialties more than others (it is most common in internal medicine and neurology) and is particularly problematic during residency training, a time of significant stress and sleep deprivation. Thankfully, discussion around mental illness has become much less "taboo" and is even encouraged, particularly in the setting of the pandemic, which has been difficult for all of us. Departments and trainees are now required to hold sessions on this topic and are encouraged to learn the warning signs of fatigue, burnout, depression, and anxiety in their trainees and students, as well as in each other.

During the pandemic, we emphasized mental health via a number of mechanisms, especially in cooperation with specific programs and offerings through the department of psychiatry. It is *not* the role of the leader to act as psychiatrist for their group or any member of it; in fact, it is likely inappropriate, although sometimes the lines are blurred when providing career counseling or discussing difficult topics. Understanding when the situation is bordering on mental illness is crucial, for at that point a professional consultation may be warranted, and the leader needs to know their boundaries. As you're keeping your finger on the pulse of the group at large, consistently trying to "read the room" and measure morale, you must also remain vigilant for the person(s) in the group who is suffering, which may be manifested by their being overly quiet or by the opposite, acting out or demonstrating behavior unusual for them.

Coming Out on the Other Side

Although at the time of writing this book our department is still in the thick of the crisis (specifically the pandemic, but also ongoing racial inequity as well as political upheaval in the US), as a leader you should always keep an eye to the future of what your group will look like when you've overcome the crisis. Everyone will crave some sense of returning to normalcy, but "normalcy" may look very different after the crisis, in both good and bad ways. Several principles may be helpful: (1) remembering what you've learned, (2) adjusting to the new normal, and (3) recalibrating the overall group goals.

Along the lines of "Never let a crisis fail to be an opportunity" make sure your group devotes some time to look back, painful as it may be, to recognize what lessons were learned, how they helped shape the group and/or its goals, and how they'll shape the group's actions in the future. You learn more from your mistakes than from your successes, and rather than wallowing in mistakes and feeling down about yourselves, use them to inform future moves and directions; further, dissect what led you to make certain mistakes and how you can grow as a thinker, planner, and doer from the experience.

Your group may not be the same after the crisis, and you'll need to adjust to the "new normal." This may be due to attrition or the addition of certain group members, or, even if all members remain, perhaps the augmentation or diminishment of the roles of some individuals. Some leaders will rise in a time of crisis, others will shrink. Conversely, some members of the group may excel in times of noncrisis. But most members will likely maintain value in one way or another, and you'll need to reestablish the group's chemistry and motivation. Part of the leader's role is taking a look at "who we are" at a given point in time, recalibrating based on internal and external factors.

Perhaps the best way to bring the group back together and recalibrate is to dig up your old mission and vision statements and reevaluate them as a group. Which goals remain, and which are new? Has the mission changed, and if so, is everyone comfortable with it and on board for next steps? What additional goals should the group take on at this time, and which ones should be eliminated? You've made it through the crisis; time to get back to a steady state but also to prepare for the next challenges your group will face!

Chapter 1

Medical Leadership 2.0

Now that you've got some core principles to rely on, let's talk about how to continue to develop as a leader. I like to think that great leadership is not something you ever really attain but rather something you are constantly striving toward. Innovation and creativity help nurture your leadership potential; resting on your laurels leads to complacency and stale leadership. This does not mean changing for the sake of change but rather always looking for ways to improve yourself and your group, keeping your eyes and ears open to potential avenues for growth and maturity.

As with all things, this does not come without some work and introspection. But I would argue that the introspection *is the work*, and most leaders fail to develop because they're unwilling or unable to take the extra steps to examine themselves and their group deeply, find out what's working and what's not, and come up with fixes.

Evaluations and Feedback

Periodic evaluations and feedback are valuable tools for continuing to develop your group and your leadership skills. These can be done in formal ways, such as yearly or biyearly 360s (see Chapter 2), or in more subtle ways, such as during weekly group or even one-on-one meetings – for example, asking the group after tackling a difficult topic, "What did everyone think of this discussion? What worked and what didn't? What were the tension points? How can we improve?" These very intentional questions, although open-ended, do send the message to your group that process improvement is important to you as a leader, both for them and for you, and that you recognize the opportunity to learn from the experience and grow.

As with all feedback, you've got to be willing to receive it. Respecting differing viewpoints is not only a means to an end (e.g. building consensus), it is validating of others and shows an openness in you to listen and learn. You will come off as less authoritarian and more group-oriented. Part of the process, however, is truly listening, even when you initially disagree with the comments of one or some group members, or worse, if you have a group member that you consciously (or subconsciously) find "annoying" or "difficult," so that you're already labeling whatever comes out of their mouth as counterproductive to the team. Effective leadership entails dealing with even those comments with respect and validation; remember, the whole group is watching you respond, and even if the group member giving the feedback does so in a negative or counterproductive way, your response does not need to be. When they go low, you go high.

When I have a one-on-one division chief or leadership meeting, I like to devote the first half of the conversation to discussing the issues within their domain and the second half to leadership development. This is bidirectional, of course, and you should always solicit feedback from them as to what is working (and not) with you as a leader, and it's a great opportunity to go over parts of their 360 evaluation with them directly. It's helpful to start with open-ended questions, such as "What were your impressions of the 360 overall? What themes do you see emerge? What did you find out about yourself? What do you think was accurate or inaccurate, and why?" And most importantly, "How do you incorporate this information and insight to improve yourself?" I find it's best in these situations to listen more and talk less. Be prepared to give your impressions, but don't start with that; allow the person to ruminate a bit and draw their own conclusions. They're much more likely to embrace change if they are the one directing the conversation and sharing their insights.

Availability, Accessibility

Although this can be challenging depending on the size of the group you're leading, I've found that one of the most successful character traits of a leader in medicine can be their accessibility and availability, especially for the core of their group. This doesn't just mean the "open door" policy, whereby some people can literally just walk into your office with an urgent issue (although this can be very useful if used sparingly!); it is also measured in responsiveness, specifically via email or other electronic means. But the rules of engagement can become blurry, and it's good to set ground rules as a group so that you're all on the same page.

I use a tiered approach in my department:

- Email – least urgent, but I will still be responsive in a reasonable timeframe. Typically less than 24 hours (usually within an hour or two during working hours). But it's helpful for the sender to tell me the timeframe in which they need the response, especially if tasks are included in the email. I eschew lengthy email chains with lots of "Thank you!" and "You're welcome!" but these are hard to avoid, and it's probably best just to use the delete button and move on.
- Text – more urgent, signals that a response is needed more promptly or perhaps giving a heads-up for a situation that may be developing. Just like

group emails (but worse!), group texts can be painful, but sometimes you can remove yourself from the text chain, often with a word to the others that you're doing so, letting them know you're no longer part of the conversation. Sometimes group members abuse texting, and this needs to be monitored, as texts are very distracting and, by definition, should command some level of importance based on urgency.

- Phone call or office drop-in – highest urgency, acute problem, you're needed right then and there. As the group leader, you may be the key problem solver, and if they need you, they need you. But if it ends up being less urgent than they thought, some education may be necessary, in a gentle way (usually).

Now, depending on your group and your personality, you may be more (or less) relaxed about these general rules, and that's fine. Find what works for you and your group, so that you're providing them with the access and responsiveness that they need to do their jobs, but you're able to maintain your sanity and can still get your work done.

Walking the Walk

There's nothing like working in clinical areas as a medical leader to give you credibility. Whether it's performing surgery, working in the ICU, taking ER shifts, working the wards, or seeing clinic patients, when your group sees you in action, they no longer see you as someone barking out orders, but as someone who is living the same experiences they are, both good and bad. So when they complain about how the clinic is dysfunctional, you can say, "I know!" and mean it! It also allows you to be part of the solution – you see things from the ground level, getting firsthand experience of the ups and downs of clinical life. However, as the leader, you should be aware that you may get hidden preferential treatment – your clinic may run better than others, as the administrative support doesn't want you to see all the problems.

Similarly, if you're leading a clinical research or educational group, you can still walk the walk. This takes the form of doing your own patient consent conversations for clinical trials, supervising resident clinic, or teaching small-group sessions. Again, this has a dual benefit – your group recognizes that you don't see yourself as "above" doing any of these things in the department, and you see for yourself what's working well and what's not. Furthermore, I find it incredibly "grounding" to participate in this way in all three realms – clinical, research, and education – this is why I went into the medical field in the first place, and I hope never to lose that passion for all of the academic missions.

Messaging

As stated multiple times throughout this book, clear, concise, and honest messaging is key. The more consistent you are with this, the more your group will trust you. Wondering and guessing are powerful and corrosive things in your group, and for whatever reason, they often go to the worst-case scenario when they lack the full picture. Maybe it's because the world is full of conspiracy theories (and those who believe them), or maybe it's just because people like to talk/gossip, and without direction they can sometimes work themselves into a frenzy. If you are able to be clear and direct with your messaging, that can help cut through all of the crap and get people to stay focused and goal-oriented.

Remember, your messaging takes several forms – directly to the group, indirectly from things they hear you reportedly said to other groups, your emails, and even your texts, tweets, and so on. Your consistency is key: if you are saying different things to different people, word gets around, and then you'll be stuck trying to explain yourself. It's best to be clear, in your own head, where you stand on an issue, and stay true to that. People expect politicians to flip-flop; they don't expect it (or tolerate it) from their medical leaders. Take your time and choose your words carefully, both oral and written.

Emails are particularly tricky, as people can't read intention or intonation; body language is, by definition, absent in written communication (although some people have learned to use emojis and tricks like that, I find them a bit unprofessional in most situations). Take your time with your emails. Be explicit and concise. Remember Strunk and White's "economy of words" – no need for flowery speech, it will just make it less likely that people will read to the end (or read it at all). And remember, once an email is sent, it can never really be retracted. A wonderful Harvard professor, Dr. Thomas Lee, once taught me: "Before you send any email, imagine what would happen if it were to fall into the worst hands possible. If there's a problem with that, then you probably shouldn't send it." Words to live by.

Embracing Change, Learning from Mistakes

This is probably the hardest trick to turn in medical leadership – using your mistakes as learning opportunities. In medicine, perhaps more than in any other profession, we are constantly striving toward perfection, as if it's always right in front of us and if we try hard enough we'll actually reach it. Of course, that's a fallacy. We're supposed to minimize morbidities and mortalities, and there is a long legacy, especially in surgical services, of raking colleagues over the coals when mistakes are made. This mindset is not only unnecessary, it is damaging to the individual and ironically likely leads to worse patient care.

Rather, an environment in which we embrace and learn from our mistakes is one in which we can truly grow and develop into better clinicians and leaders. And I would argue that it needs to come from the top of the food chain – typically the group's leader needs to be the first to say, "I was wrong and here is why." If the leader is able to lead by example, embracing humility and the spirit of education and quality improvement, others will feel empowered and motivated to share their thoughts (and fears) as well. And when the leader recognizes that a more junior member of the group is sticking their neck out, at some risk, it is important that the leader applaud the act, recognizing the bravery for the group, even celebrating it. I will often say something like "That must have taken a lot of guts for you to have said that, and we thank you!" If these are the first words that come out of the group leader's mouth when a mistake has been made, the table has been set for an inclusive, respectful environment that embraces learning from mistakes.

The other thing a leader can applaud is innovation and change. It is very easy to fall into a rut or routine; in fact, there's a level of comfort in it. But change and new ideas are necessary for any group, and in medicine it's important that we challenge dogma when it doesn't make sense (perhaps it made sense in another era, but not now). Doing my residency in the 1990s, I never challenged dogma . . . and there was a lot of it where I trained. But it was only when I started to question the "principles" that lacked an evidence base that I truly started to grow as a clinician, and it planted the roots for me to become a leader. I didn't realize it at the time, but I was entering a rite of passage, similar to when your child leaves the nest; challenging dogma was a necessity if I was ever to grow as a clinician and leader. My job now is to create an environment for clinicians (and administrators) in my own department to celebrate change and innovation every time it happens; people should not be ashamed of coming up with new ideas and solutions, but rather congratulated for it (even if their ideas don't pan out).

Embracing Diversity

Another running theme in this book is diversity. Recognizing that diversity takes on many forms and definitions, from the perspective of your group's success, diversity in medicine should include representation (of the larger group, which can include the patient population, the institution/school, or both), perspective (people who can look at things from different angles than you and others in the group), experience (what do people bring to the table, including their gender, race, ethnicity, sexual orientation, and life experiences), and personality. From a personality standpoint, it may be tempting to pick people to join your group who think like you, act like you, talk like you, and look like you; however, those groups will likely become stagnant, lack innovation, and never become high achievers. The days of the "good ole boys club" are dying (thankfully); the more successful groups have learned to diversify in order to grow, mature, and reach greater heights.

Core Features

You may or may not want to do this, but I find it helpful to distill my leadership skills down into some core features or principles. Think of it as an informal, simplistic 360 you can do on yourself periodically, maybe once a year. What are the things that make you special as a leader? What are the strengths that you can play to and inspire others to emulate? What traits or characteristics that you currently lack might be beneficial for you to incorporate into your persona, with some work?

If I had to distill my most effective leadership traits down to five, I would list integrity, fairness, compassion, transparency, and respect. Sure, these are lofty words, and there are probably others that I might consider putting on the list as well. But there are probably many more that are *not* on that list that should be, traits that, if I were able to incorporate them, would be highly beneficial to my leadership. (Lest you think me completely unhumble, these would include patience, decreased volatility, and a thicker skin, to name a few!) As leaders, we should all be aware of what makes us effective, as well as our Achilles' heels. Taking the time to take stock of both is a useful periodic exercise. Not all leaders will have the same core features (good or bad); understanding yours will make you a more effective leader.

"3 Ps": Patience, Positivity, Perseverance

I will close with the principle that has guided me as I've emerged as a leader in medicine, the "3 Ps": patience, positivity, and perseverance. More than anything else, these three friends have been a compass and guide, especially in difficult times. As a medical leader, you will undoubtedly experience challenges and difficult times; *because* you are leader, you are expected to guide your group through them.

Patience. You will not fix everything overnight, and most (not all) problems for your medical group will take some time to figure out and come to a workable solution; the more complex the problem, the more patient you will need to be. Quick fixes usually don't last; group fixes, worked through with time and patience, stand a much better chance.

Positivity. It sounds simplistic, but if you're able to remain positive no matter what is going on around you, you are bound to be successful as a leader in medicine. If you're positive, people will naturally gravitate toward your leadership much more than if you're sour, complaining, or dictatorial (most people like positive people, especially when they're feeling insecure themselves). Positivity is infectious, and the more you're able to convey yours, the more positive your group will become. The creativity will blossom, the work ethic will increase, and the productivity will soar. Maintaining a positive culture in medical groups is a hidden key to success.

Perseverance. Even if you're the most positive and patient person on the planet, if you're unable to persevere through adversity, your group will not succeed. When (not "if") you hit roadblocks, your leadership is what will bring the group through to the other side. Helping them to understand that sometimes things don't come easily, but the goals are worth the sacrifice, allows them to maintain their faith in you and rise to the challenges. If you give up, so will they. If you persevere, they will be inspired, and the end result (hopefully by overcoming the obstacles) will be that much more rewarding since you had to work for it. You came through it together, as a group. And now you're ready to handle anything!

Appendix 1 BU Neurology Vision Statement 2020

The Neurology Department at Boston University School of Medicine (BUSM) and Boston Medical Center (BMC) will lead the field in advancing the care of patients with neurological disease through the best clinical care, innovative research and the education of tomorrow's leaders in Neurology in a culture that embodies diversity, inclusion, equity, critical thinking, and innovation.

Core Areas

- **Culture** – the culture of the department should reflect its core values, including:

    - Putting the patient at the center of everything we do
    - Creating and maintaining an environment of equity, vitality, and inclusion
    - Respect for all others, regardless of their role/position or identity
    - Emphasis on wellness and vitality
    - Embracing diversity for the true value that it can bring to our department, enabling us to grow and mature responsibly and with a strong moral compass
    - Teamwork to improve care and morale

- **Clinical** – we will fulfill BMC's overall mission of "Exceptional Care Without Exception" by providing the best care possible, regardless of a patient's means, background, or socioeconomic status.

- **Research** – exceptional research throughout the department, including basic science, translational, and clinical research.

- **Education** – continuing the tradition of excellence of neurological education established through our history as Boston City Hospital, Boston University Hospital, and Boston Medical Center.

- **Administration (Operations and Finances)** – establishing a well-run department from an administrative standpoint, including efficient outpatient and inpatient operations that enable excellent clinical care and high productivity from providers.

Metrics

- **Culture**

    - Reputation – as measured by Doximity, others
    - US News and World Report ranking
    - Wellness surveys within our department
    - Programs and committees focused on wellness, diversity, and inclusion

- ○ Recruiting and retaining excellent faculty, including from a wide range of gender, race, ethnicity, and other backgrounds
- ○ Eliminating any and all forms of racism, discrimination, and harassment
- ○ Teamwork – ability to form functional, high-performing teams, both within neurology and with other departments

- **Clinical**

  - ○ Outcomes – by disease state, compared with national benchmarks, stratified by age, race, gender, socioeconomic status, and other variables
  - ○ Patient satisfaction survey results, compared with BMC, regional and national benchmarks
  - ○ Provide comprehensive clinical care by establishing and using state-of-the-art diagnostic tools and novel therapies to improve patient outcomes
  - ○ Innovation in clinical care – novel therapies that lead to improved patient outcomes and dissemination of results for others to model
  - ○ "Top Doctor" awards, both locally and nationally
  - ○ Establish and maintain centers of excellence in key clinical areas (e.g. Multiple Sclerosis, Epilepsy, Stroke, Sleep, Pain)
  - ○ Develop metrics of success based on division/domain
  - ○ Referrals in vs. referrals out for specialized treatment

- **Research**

  - ○ All divisions/specialties have annual publications in high-impact journals
  - ○ Lead principal investigator-initiated multicenter clinical trials
  - ○ Provide structure and support for junior faculty to pursue research interests
  - ○ Innovation in research leading to impactful novel discoveries
  - ○ NIH and extramural funding of high quality research
  - ○ Total number of publications by individual faculty and the department as a whole
  - ○ Cross-disciplinary collaboration
  - ○ Research awards, both locally and nationally

- **Education**

  - ○ Teaching evaluations by students and residents, compared with BMC, regional and national benchmarks
  - ○ Innovation in education, leading to publication or other dissemination (e.g. lectures, symposia, courses)
  - ○ Resident surveys compared with BMC, regional and national benchmarks

- ○ CME courses by each division
- ○ Publications in neurologic educational research
- ○ Education awards, both locally and nationally

- **Administration (Operations and Finances)**

  - ○ Financial productivity (actual vs. budget)
  - ○ RVU generation toward goal metrics based on the individual's role
  - ○ Provider satisfaction with work processes
  - ○ Staff satisfaction with work processes
  - ○ Adequate and appropriate administrative staffing
  - ○ Maintain and sustain a competitive compensation plan
  - ○ Attract philanthropy and grow endowed funds to $XX million
  - ○ All divisions/specialties have new patient appointment availability within 2 weeks (or some other metrics for access)
  - ○ Embrace and encourage a diverse leadership (gender, race, etc.)

Resources

Please find below a short list of potentially helpful resources for your reading list as a leader. Some of these are from the business world, others from medicine; some may be for your initial time as a leader, others for maintenance and growth after you've been on the job for a while.

- Patrick Lencioni, *The Five Dysfunctions of a Team* (San Francisco: Jossey-Bass, 2002)
- Thomas Neff and James Citrin, "Now You're In Charge: The First 100 Days" (April 2004), www.spencerstuart.com/research-and-insight/now-youre-in-charge-the-first-100-days
- Roselinde Torres and Peter Tollman, "Five myths of a CEO's first 100 days," *Harvard Business Review* (January 30, 2012), https://hbr.org/2012/01/five-myths-of-a-ceos-first-100
- Peter Tollman and Roselinde Torres, "Debunking the Myths of the First 100 Days" (January 3, 2013), www.bcg.com/publications/2013/people-organization-leadership-talent-debunking-myths-first-100-days
- Merete Wedell-Wedellsborg, "How to lead when your team is exhausted – and you are too," *Harvard Business Review* (December 15, 2020), https://hbr.org/2020/12/how-to-lead-when-your-team-is-exhausted-and-you-are-too
- Michael D. Watkins, *HBR's 10 Must Reads for New Managers* (Boston, MA: Harvard Business Publishing, 2017)
- Stephen R. Covey, *The 7 Habits of Highly Effective People: Powerful Lessons in Personal Change* (San Francisco: FranklinCovey, 2016)
- Rasmus Hougaard and Jacqueline Carter, *The Mind of the Leader: How to Lead Yourself, Your People, and Your Organization for Extraordinary Results* (Boston, MA: Harvard Business School Publishing, 2018)
- Mike Krzyzewski, *Leading with the Heart* (New York: Warner, 2001)
- Ken Blanchard and Spencer Johnson, *The New One Minute Manager* (London: HarperCollins Publishers, 2015)
- Daniel Coyle, *The Culture Code: The Secrets of Highly Successful Groups* ([n.p.]: Bantam Books, 2018)
- Daniel James Brown, *The Boys in the Boat: An Epic Journey to the Heart of Hitler's Berlin* (London: Pan Books, 2014)
- Robert Greene, *The Laws of Human Nature* (New York: Viking, 2018)

- Manasa S. Ayyala et al., "Mentorship is not enough: Exploring sponsorship and its role in career advancement in academic medicine," *Academic Medicine*, 94 (2019): 94–100

- Project Management Institute, *A Guide to the Project Management Body of Knowledge (PMBOK Guide)*, 5th ed. (Newton Square, PA: Project Management Institute, 2013)

- Tasha Eurich, *Insight: The Surprising Truth about How Others See Us, How We See Ourselves, and Why the Answers Matter More Than We Think* (New York: Currency, 2018)

- Douglas Stone, Bruce Patton, and Sheila Heen, *Difficult Conversations, How to Discuss What Matters Most* (London: Penguin, 2000)

- John Doerr, *Measure What Matters: How Google, Bono, and the Gates Foundation Rock the World with OKRs* (New York: Portfolio/Penguin, 2018)

- Michael D. Watkins, *The First 90 Days: Proven Strategies for Getting Up to Speed Faster and Smarter* (Boston, MA: Harvard Business School Publishing, 2013)

- Jocko Willink and Leif Babin, *The Dichotomy of Leadership: Balancing the Challenges of Extreme Ownership to Lead and Win* (New York: St Martin's Press, 2018)

- Doris Kearns Goodwin, *Team of Rivals: The Political Genius of Abraham Lincoln* (New York: Simon & Schuster, 2005)

- Jonathan Raymond, *Good Authority: How to Become the Leader Your Team Is Waiting For* ([n.p.]: Idea Press, 2016)

- Renate B. Schnabel and Emelia J. Benjamin, "Diversity 4.0 in the cardiovascular health-care workforce," *Nature Reviews Cardiology*, 17 (December 2020): 751–3

- Myers-Briggs Type Indicator: www.mbtionline.com

- DISC Personality Profile: www.discpersonalitytesting.com

Index